SWITCHING ON

A Guide to Edu-Kinesthetics™

By Paul E. Dennison, Ph.D.

Published by

Edu-Kinesthetics, Inc.
P.O. Box 3396
Ventura, CA 93006-3396
(805) 650-3303

Copyright © 1981
by
Paul E. Dennison, Ph.D.

Third Edition

All rights reserved. No part of this book may be reproduced in any form or by any means without the prior written permission of the publisher.

TO
LAURIE
VALERIE
and
THOMAS

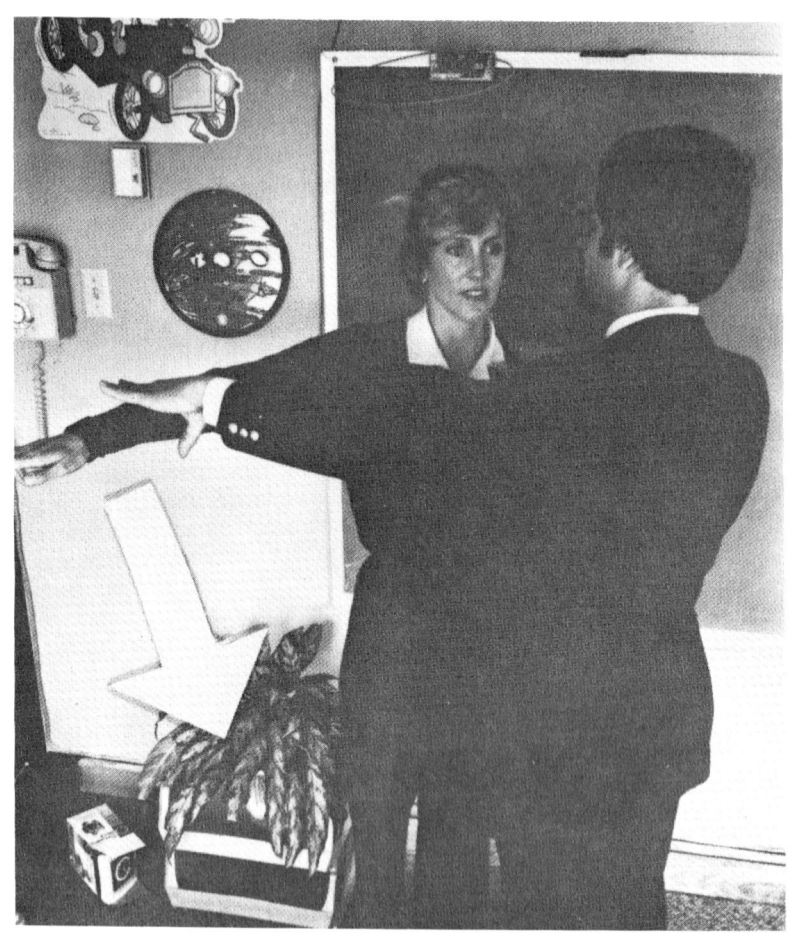

Fig. 1. Testing the deltoid muscle of your partner.

YOU CAN DO THIS!

Before you read this book, perform the following exercise with your partner:

1. Stand facing your partner as illustrated in Figure 1.

2. Ask your partner to lift his arm to shoulder height, keeping the other relaxed at his side.

3. Place your hand on his outstretched arm, just above the wrist, and rest your other hand on his opposite shoulder to place him at ease.

4. Tell your partner that when you give the signal to "hold," you will press his arm down towards the floor. His job is to hold his arm up and prevent you from doing so.

5. Say, "Hold," as you firmly press his arm down. You are pressing just hard enough to feel a muscle "switch on" and lock the shoulder joint against the pressure.

6. Thank your partner for cooperating so well. Did you feel the muscle get switched on? In nearly every case this muscle is easy to lock.

Now add the following variation. Repeating steps 1 through 4 above, when you get to step number 5 and are saying "Hold," add:
"Try your hardest." "Try your best."
Was his response the same, or different? Did the muscle switch on or switch off this time? Invariably, the thought of "trying hard" will make it more difficult to lock the muscle and his arm can easily be pressed to his side.

Now add the following variation after preparing your partner for the muscle test. After you say "Hold," add:
"You can do this. Be the best you can be!"
How did the muscle feel now? Did the muscle switch on, or switch off? Invariably, he will do as well, or even better than the first time with this simple encouragement to be himself.

Why did the little word "try" produce a **different response?** You are reading this book to learn the answer.

ACKNOWLEDGEMENTS

The author has been blessed throughout his life with hundreds of loving guides who believed in him, showed him the path, and always stood by him. Without listing individual names, for they know who they are, love and energy is radiated to them, one and all.

TABLE OF CONTENTS

Preface 6
Foreword by Richard H. Tyler, D.C. 7
Chapter I. Introduction—What is Edu-Kinesthetics? 11
Chapter II. Muscle Testing 14
  —The Importance of Touch 14
  —Preparing Yourself for Muscle Testing 15
  —What is Muscle Testing? 16
  —What is an Indicator Muscle? 17
  —How Do You Test a Muscle? 17
  —Preparing Another for Muscle Testing 18
  —The Muscles 19

Chapter III. Energy and The Environment 24
  —What Is Color? 24
  —Sound and Music 25
  —Food and Our Energy Fields 26
  —The Power of Words 27
  —Natural vs. Plastic 28
  —Television 28
  —People 28

Chapter IV. Stress and Negative Thinking 30
  —Reducing Stress 31
  —Procedure for Emotional Stress Release 32

Chapter V. Cross-Motor Patterning 35
  —Dyslexia and Learning Disabilities 35
  —What is Cross-Motor Patterning? 37
  —Who Needs Cross-Crawling? 40
  —Teaching and Learning Suggestions 42
  —Evaluation of Results 44

Chapter VI. Posture From Within 48
  —The Neck Is Critical 49
  —Balance Dimensions 49
  —Reprogramming Energy Flow 50
  —Movement Re-Education 53
  —Postural Analysis 55

Chapter VII.	Lateral Dominance	57
	—Handedness and Eyedness	57
	—Brainedness and Eye Movements	61
	—Technique to Determine the Dominant Brain	63
	—Visual Integration	63
	—Edu-Kinesthetics and the Ears	70
	—Dennison Laterality Checklist	75
Chapter VIII.	Prologue—Two Extreme Opposites— Brain Left and Brain Right	76
	A Switched-on Brain	79
	—The Human Brain	80
	—Jimmy and the Midline	83
	—Two Learning Types	87
	—Characteristics of Left and Right Brain	89
Chapter IX.	Writing Analysis	91
	—Handedness and Writing Ability	93
	—Counterclockwise Energy	94
	—The "Lazy 8"	94
	—Posture and Writing	96
Chapter X.	Switch On to Reading	99
	—Traditional Educational Procedures	100
	—Fred, a True Dyslexic	101
	—Grace, a Stroke Victim	102
Chapter XI.	E-K in Action	105
	—The Poseidon School	105
	—An Educational Philosophy	105
	—Staff Development	106
	—Accountability	106
	—The Classroom	106
	—The Students	107
	—Results	107
	—Our Symbol	111
Definition of Terms		112
Appendix: Edu-Exercises		113
Bibliography		118
Index		120

PREFACE

American education is in a state of crisis. Learning disabilities abound in every school. Tens of millions of functional illiterates have been passed through the system, and their numbers are growing fast. Students in general are losing the capacity for written and verbal expression, as well as common mathematical computation. Even the competence of teachers is being challenged as we enter the Eighties.

The Department of Education says that three percent of American children, or about two million youngsters, have learning disabilities. Experts in the field suggest figures that are much higher—perhaps ten to twelve million, ranging from those under-achievers, who fail when they could succeed as top students, to the severely educationally handicapped.

This book tells *why* we are in the present educational dilemma, and *how* we can get out of it. The techniques included are based on the latest discoveries in experimental psychology and brain research in America, yet they also confirm our most ancient perceptions of how we learn and grow.

Learning problems are not diseases. They are "crossed wires" in the communication network which connects a child to his world. The learning disabled child has a "jammed system," because he has been *switched off* by today's high pressure, competitive approach to education. The wonderful irony is how easily we can *switch on* our frustrated children to the exciting adventure learning is meant to be.

Switching On is a manual of hope for the concerned parents and frustrated teachers of the "unteachable" child. Used with love and confidence, these simple techniques bring results in amazingly little time. They represent a revolutionary new approach to learning.

For the adult who might have experienced a traumatic childhood or learned to hate school, *Switching On* offers a second chance. It is never too late to get "switched-on" to the joy that learning adds to life.

FOREWORD

Very early in the educational process of my son, I found that he wasn't learning to read. Maybe he was just a bit slow, we rationalized. As time went by, however, it became increasingly apparent that he wasn't making any progress, but was still being passed into higher grades by the school. Conferences with the teachers proved worthless and frustration grew with time. In exasperation, we had I.Q. tests given, and found out that our son was an average boy, with full capacity to learn. He had the "tools," but apparently wasn't being instructed how to use them.

Fortunately, I was practicing in a building at the time that had, in one of the offices, a specialist in developing the learning acuity of both children and adults. In an exercise of desperation, I brought my son to the therapist, Paul Dennison, Ph.D. After extensive testing, it was discovered that my son had dyslexia, a condition in which the individual experiences difficulty in reading, due to a diminished perceptual coordination. After months of concerted training in the proper method of reading, he returned to his studies, and went to the head of the class. This taught us a lesson, and when one of our daughters displayed the signs of dyslexia, we went once again to Dr. Dennison, with the same positive results.

Over the years, my regard for Dr. Dennison grew as I would watch those I would send to him experience the value of his teaching.

Another thing that impressed me was his unusual intellectual dedication to the purpose of what he was doing. He never seemed satisfied. He felt that he was laboring against some kind of invisible wall, and delighted that he achieved results in spite of it. If only there were some way of breaking through that wall, instead of having to climb over it.

Dr. Dennison was a patient of mine, and after a while, he began to question the possibility of there being a connection between body mechanics and perceptual distress. Was it possible that some kind of muscular imbalance might act as a handicap to the mechanics of reading? He was particularly interested in my use of applied kinesiology. It intrigued him to see muscles that might test weak respond to the light touch techniques of reflexology. As the years went by, he catalogued the concepts of reflexology, but never knew how to apply them to his work.

After taking courses in muscle balancing techniques, Dr. Dennison felt he held the key to what he was seeking. He decided to muscle test one of his students. Before doing anything, he had him hold his head still while following a moving object with his eyes. As usual, when the student tracked from one side to the other, there was a point of apparent confusion when he reached the midpoint. It was an "invisible wall" that the eyes couldn't seem to pass. Dennison then had the pupil perform a cross-crawl by lifting one arm and the opposite leg in alternate moves for several repetitions. Once again he tried the tracking test with the eyes, and this time the wall seemed to have vanished. With controlled anticipation, he tested the student's reading acuity, and was impressed with the relative eagerness with which the young man now seemed to respond to the challenge of the reading assignments and perceptual tests.

In the months that followed, Dennison increased the scope of his muscle testing procedures, and began to keep a detailed account of the areas of weakness and the response obtained from the reflexology. It was at this point that he called to tell me of his research. He felt that it would be in the best interests of what he was trying to achieve for his students to have a physical examination and muscle evaluation given by a chiropractic physician.

I proceeded to work with him for several months. The work was exciting and emotionally rewarding, as we would seemingly "unlock" people from the bonds of perceptual handicaps. Using his Edu-Kinesthetics, Dr. Dennison soon found that he could help all people, whatever their learning goals might be. Considering the fantastic capabilities of the human mind, the most incredible computer ever conceived, we are all "learning handicapped," and are unaware of our true potential. If we are only using ten percent of our minds (and we are probably using even less than that), then we are certainly imprisoned by some switching-off mechanism. If you want to break through the wall to the unlimited expansion of your potential, or if you want to "switch on" yourself and your loved ones to a better life, I recommend a careful reading of this book.

Richard A. Tyler, D.C.
June, 1981

POEM
(Recited by Goldie Hawn, written by Digby Wolfe)

Here's to the kids who are different;
The kids who don't always get "A's,"
The kids who have ears
twice the size of their peers,
or have noses that go on for days.

Here's to the kids who are different;
The kids who are just out of step,
The kids they all tease,
Who have cuts on their knees,
And whose sneakers are constantly wet.

Here's to the kids who are different;
The kids with a mischievous streak,
For when they have grown,
As history has shown,
It's their differences that make them unique.

CHAPTER I
INTRODUCTION
WHAT IS EDU-KINESTHETICS?

Edu-Kinesthtics, or E-K, is an invaluable tool for parents and teachers. It is a unique merging of applied kinesiology and learning theory to facilitate learning and eliminate uncertainty as one guides another's growth. By understanding how "Energy" can be blocked and released, one improves not only his learning, but the quality of his life as well.

Applied Kinesiology has provided a new perspective on teaching and learning. Kinesiology is the study of muscles, and the science of testing and balancing them to restore equilibrium. Applied Kinesiology means that we apply the information that the muscles can tell us about the mind and body to facilitate our work.

Most of the knowledge upon which Edu-Kinesthetics is based is of ancient origin. George Goodheart, D.C., is credited with much of the innovation known as "muscle testing." John F. Thie, D.C., author of *Touch for Health*, has synthesized this information for the layman. The application of kinesiology to education is the result of research by the author at Valley Remedial Group, a learning center in California.

Edu-Kinesthetics should not be confused with Psycho-Motor Training. These two approaches share the same goals— improved health and learning ability through balance and coordination. They are different, however. Edu-Kinesthetics include some psycho-motor exercises, but it eliminates most of them as redundant. Edu-Kinesthetics is not a "method," but rather a tool for making any system for teaching work better.

In Edu-Kinesthetics, the body and the mind are viewed as one. The posture of an individual is his "body English." If we allow ourselves to read what a person is telling us with his body, we can understand him better. As we understand the brain and the learning process, we can get even more clues from observing each other. Intervention to improve the posture through Applied Kinesiology and exercises makes all learning easier as unnecessary stress is eliminated. That is the most exciting part!

Our philosophy has been one which accepts the learner as a unique, growing, good person who will learn when given a nurturing environment.

We have generally avoided labeling and categorizing people as being "learning disabled," "dyslexic," etc., a practice consistent with the medical profession's treatment of disease. Instead, we have sought to help our students develop fully, integrating sensory modes so that they learn to function as whole individuals.

Believing the principle of growth to apply to our staff, as well, we have encouraged our therapists to be creative and suggest, but never insist that one methodology is superior to any other. We believe that there are many "right" methods within the framework of our philosophy.

Each child learns differently and is as unlike any other as are two fingerprints. The skillful teacher will have many methods and ideas to help fit a therapeutic approach to the diagnosis. As the child grows, the diagnosis must change with him. It is never static.

We have been eclectic over the years, gleaning information and ideas from many sources. Our therapy utilizes techniques borrowed from languages specialists, optometrists, and chiropractors. In a search for alternatives, we have had to go beyond the educational frame of reference.

Our philosophy is to be aware of, and to do what works. These techniques have been successful for us. We have helped children gain three years' academic growth in one. We have seen I.Q. scores soar and personalities change. We have helped to make "I cannot" into "I can!" We will continue to seek new and better methods to accomplish our goals, while refining and improving upon the knowledge of the past.

Before going any further in this book, pose these questions to yourself:

"What is my philosophy of education?"
"What do I think is the responsibility of our schools?"
Make some notes to set aside; then reread them when you complete the book.

If you had some difficulty expressing your concept of how we learn, you are not alone, for these problems have inspired poets and philosophers for centuries. The confusion comes because we have all been conditioned by a system which rewards objective, verbal, linear thinking. Our concept of intelligence has been based upon logical, rational, and scientific abilities. Intelligence tests reward such thinking with high scores, and our modern technological society has been built in this image. This mode of consciousness is left-brain thinking, and we have all been taught that we must excel in this area.

This book will give you a new perspective upon learning, without denying the validity of any of the above. It will seek to show the importance of a high "right-brain" I.Q. and how to achieve a right-brain/left-brain balance through touch, movement, posture, breathing, and love.

CHAPTER II
MUSCLE TESTING

The Importance of Touch

Edu-Kinesthetics utilizes muscle testing as a diagnostic and therapeutic tool to get in tune with our natural body energy. The muscle testing requires that we touch each other, which even by itself is extremely beneficial.

Our modern American culture has drifted so completely into multi-media information processing that we have forgotten how to touch and feel. Our language is replete with visual and auditory figures of speech, such as, "I see the point," "I hear what you are saying," and "I'll look into it." We seldom talk about feelings, and even though we ask, "How are you?" we don't know how to react to any other answer but "Fine."

Touching has been proven necessary for normal physical and mental development. Hospitals employ women whose job it is to pick up, cuddle, and handle infants if the mother is not available. Breast feeding and other physical stimulation by mothers has been proven to produce significantly higher I.Q.'s than when less touching has been provided.

Our society has conditioned us that touch is reserved for either punitive or sexual encounters. There is a bumper sticker that reads, "Have You Hugged Your Child Today?" Do parents really have to be reminded to love their children? Many children will misbehave, preferring a spanking to being ignored physically. How many young people are so hungry for touch that they enter into sexual encounters for which they are not emotionally prepared?

A friend of ours looks forward to his monthly hairstyling because he enjoys the feeling of the operator giving him a shampoo! We go to doctors and chiropractors, often just for the touching care. Touching makes us feel better. Edu-Kinesthetics will help to explain why.

When we touch and muscle test each other, we are entering a person's life space. Pretend that there is an eighteen inch or so layer surrounding you and your partner. When you enter that space, you enter his Energy field and mix your Energy and his. Your Energy affects his, and his affects yours. This can be demonstrated with muscle testing. If you will remember to prepare yourself for touching encounters, you will have positive experiences that are understood by both you and your partner.

Preparing Yourself For Muscle Testing

Edu-Kinesthetics suggests that you prepare yourself for muscle testing another by:

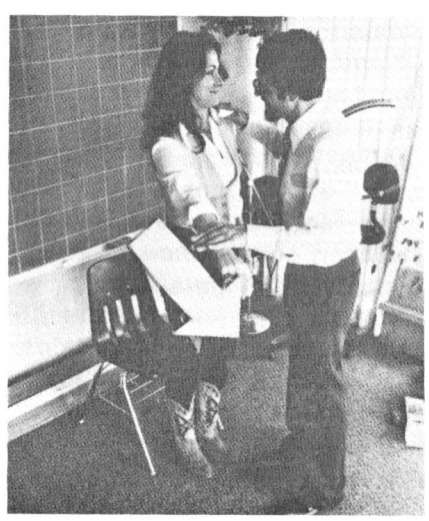

Fig 1. Testing the supraspinatus muscle.

1. achieving your own state of balance physically, emotionally, and spiritually through E-K techniques, which you will learn throughout this book;

2. assuming a posture of unconditional love and intention to help the person to be tested;

3. assuming a posture of centeredness where you will shield and protect your own Energy field from any negativity that the person to be tested might transmit to you;

4. assuming an attitude of loving detachment where you will not expect any particular response from your subject other than the response his body will give.

WHAT IS MUSCLE TESTING?

Muscle testing is the art of isolating and testing one muscle at a time in order to determine if it is weak or strong, relative to the strength of the individual being tested. The purpose is to detect Energy imbalance. The question is, has something happened to "switch off" the muscle? The language, "weak" and "strong," is used when testing muscles. When we say this, we mean "switched-off" or "switched-on." Muscles test "weak" only because there is a short circuit in the Energy signal from the brain to the muscle. We will learn many possible causes for such interruptions in Energy flow. Remember for now, that when we test muscles, we are testing Energy, not physical strength.

Our research at Valley Remedial Group has shown us that certain select muscles, which you will easily learn to test, provide us with all the information we need to teach each other. Children and adults with learning disabilities show Energy blockages when these muscles are tested. In most cases, when these muscles are strengthened through E-K techniques, academic performance dramatically improves.

Muscle testing is both safe and simple. A muscle is either strong or weak. There is no arbitrary judgment made by an authority figure. The learner feels the weak muscle. He also feels the strengthening process. There is both an advantage for the evaluator who is diagnosing, and for the learner who is experiencing the process of change, feeling the balancing, feeling his coordination return, and preparing himself to learn.

WHAT IS AN INDICATOR MUSCLE?

Every muscle test indicates or tells us something. The *intention* of a muscle test is very important. When we test a muscle, we are asking the body and Energy field a question. For example, when we test the Supraspinatus muscle, we are asking the body if there is Energy blockage involved with mental fatigue. When we test the Pectoralis Major Clavicular muscle, we are asking the body if there is Energy blockage in regard to emotional stress. When we test the Latissimus Dorsi, we are asking the body about sugar metabolism and food allergies. Any muscle can be used when we ask the body questions. A good muscle to use, because it is usually strong and readily accessible without throwing the body off balance, both in a standing and sitting position, is the Deltoid. (See Figure 2 for the location of the muscles on the body.)

HOW DO YOU TEST A MUSCLE?

To test a muscle, we apply pressure *in the opposite direction* from the way the muscle moves when it works. For example, the Deltoid muscle is located in the shoulder and lifts the arm up when it contracts. Feel and try it on yourself. Put one hand on your shoulder and lift your arm straight up. Feel the shoulder tighten and shorten as your arm rises. Now hold arm in the "up" position. The muscle test for the Deltoid would involve pressure to move the arm down again while you resist or hold it in the "up" position. You may test the muscle anywhere within its "range of motion." Choose a position comfortable for you and your partner.

When you test a muscle, you are not trying to overpower it. You are feeling for the *ability to "lock" the muscle.* Does the muscle feel "switched-off" or "switched-on"? The main problem in learning muscle testing is overpowering with too much pressure. Except for those of very large body-builders, all muscles can be overpowered, especially those of children. So feel for a locking sensation, and let go. The steps to follow to test the four muscles in Figure 2 are:

1. Demonstrate the range of motion of the isolated muscle by moving the arm up and down in the direction in which the muscle works.

2. Rehearse the test by saying, "I am going to press your arm this way. You hold it here and do not let me do it."
3. Test the muscle by saying, "Ready, hold it!"
4. Use the 2-2-2 technique. Test with two fingers and an open palm. Hold the pressure for two seconds. If the muscle (arm) moves two inches, it is weak.
5. Record your findings. (For example, Right Supraspinatus locks, or Deltoid weak)

PREPARING ANOTHER FOR MUSCLE TESTING

We have already discussed how to prepare yourself for muscle testing another. To prepare your subject, it is important to explain what you are going to do and why you are doing it. The points to remember to discuss are:

1. Does he know of any reason why a muscle test is inadvisable? It is better to ask beforehand than to be surprised.
2. He is in control of the testing. If anything should cause pain or discomfort, he is to signal loudly and clearly so that the testing will stop.
3. You are looking for his ability to hold the muscle. You are not trying to overpower him or engage in a "tug of war." You are working together to discover energy imbalances. Invite his cooperation and keep it fun.

Now turn to Chapter 3 and do some muscle testing right away. It is really quite simple. The position for testor and testee are illustrated in Figures 3, 4, 5, 6.

The range of motion follows the direction of the testor's left hand (see arrows). Remember that you do not move the arm through the whole range of motion when testing. If it is "switched-off" for *two* inches, it is weak. It is a good idea to rest one hand on the opposite shoulder as you test, to both relax and assure the testee as you press on his arm.

"TOUCH FOR HEALTH"

For more information on muscle testing, made simple for the layperson, I recommend "Touch For Health," by John F. Thie, D.C. Dr. Thie provides a complete program for muscle balancing through touch techniques.

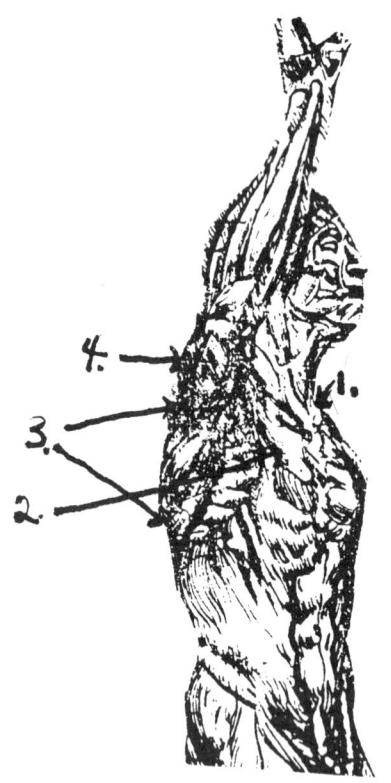

Fig. 2

THE MUSCLES
  The four mucles used in Edu-Kinesthetics are:
1. Supraspinatus
2. Pectoralis Major Clavicular
3. Latissimus Dorsi
4. Deltoid

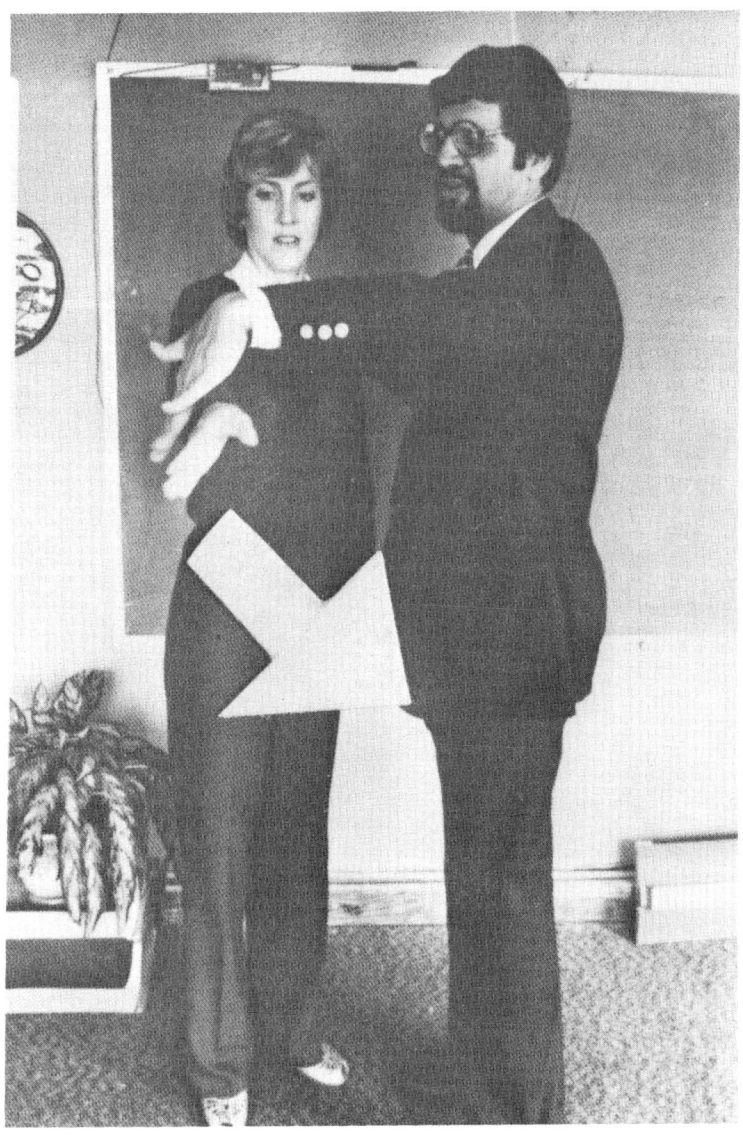

Fig. 3. Testing the supraspinatus muscle. Press down and towards the midline of the body (See arrow for the direction).

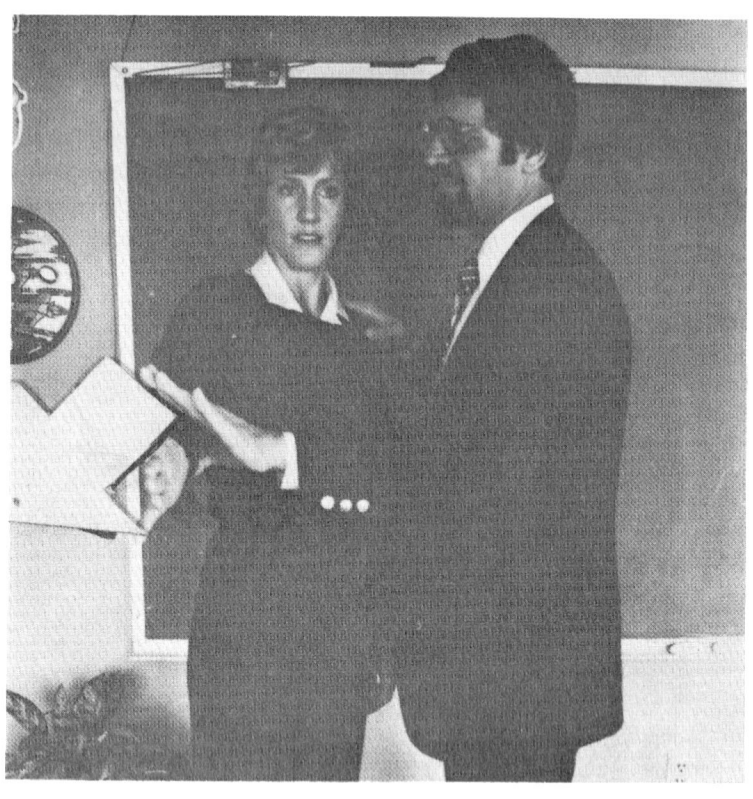

Fig. 4. Testing the pectoralis major clavicular muscle. Press down and away from the body (See arrow for the direction).

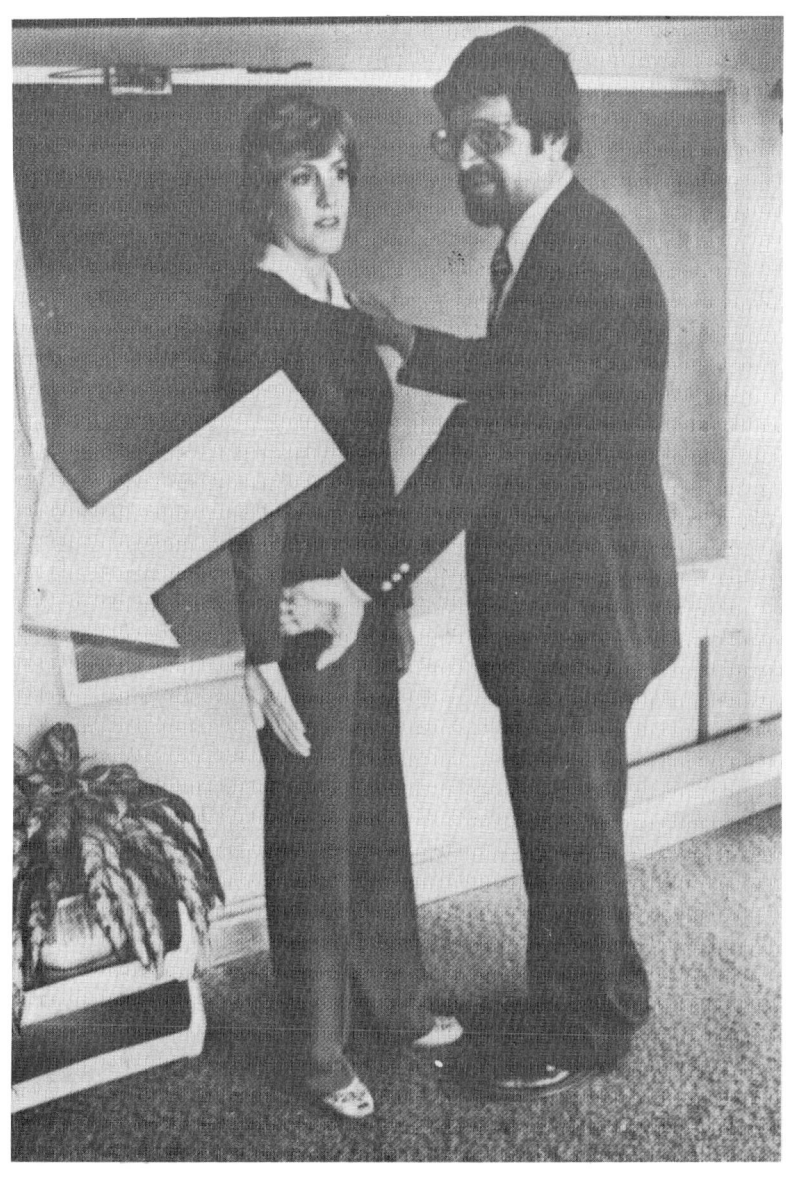

Fig. 5. Testing the latissimus dorsi muscle. Your partner turns his hand so that the palm faces away from the body. While he holds it against his body, as if it were "glued to his hip," you attempt to pull it away from the body.

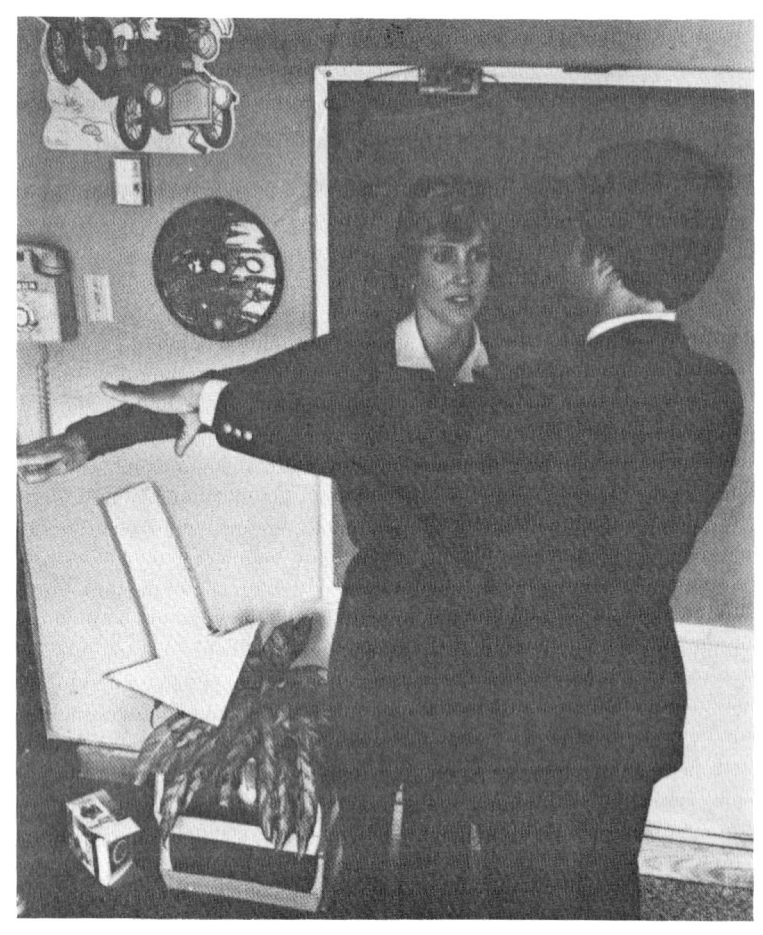

Fig. 6. Testing the deltoid muscle. Press down towards the side of the body.

CHAPTER III
ENERGY AND THE ENVIRONMENT

The previous chapter discussed muscle testing and introduced the concept of Energy flowing in our Lifespace. We learned to test certain muscles, and we learned that a weak muscle meant Energy blockage somewhere in the system. In this chapter, we will learn more about Energy, and we will see demonstrated, as well as experience, that we are all, at a certain level, Energy, and are therefore subject to environmental influences beyond our conscious, rational control.

As we learn about Energy, active participation is mandatory. Many books have been written on the subject, yet few people understand this force. Call it Chi, Prana, Cosmic Energy, or Love; people have accepted its existence on faith, while only a few have felt it and used it successfully. Muscle testing enables even the most skeptical to experience something of its power. It is not necessary to understand what is happening. Only feel what we experience as muscles switch on and off, and we will recognize that something is taking place. That will be enough to make Edu-Kinesthetics work for us.

WHAT IS COLOR?
We live in a world filled with color. People talk about their favorite colors. "Red makes me sick." "I hate blue." "Green is my favorite color." What is it about certain colors that affects our moods and our ability to concentrate?

Color is Energy vibrating at different frequencies. Different colors influence Energy fields in different ways. There are

Energy centers within our bodies which are tuned into different Energy frequencies. Certain frequencies help to achieve Energy balance for the whole body. Other frequencies concentrate energy and the overload results in switching off.

Do some muscle testing with colors to learn its effect on your own Energy. Work with a partner. Use any indicator muscle. The Deltoid is excellent for the purpose.

STEPS FOR MUSCLE TESTING FOR COLOR AND OTHER ENVIRONMENTAL FACTORS
1. First test the indicator muscle to verify if it is strong. This is called "testing in the clear."
2. Select the environmental factor to be tested.
3. Ask your subject to concentrate upon the factor. For example, "Look at the color pink in Fran's blouse." (Most objects may be held in the hand, or touched.)
4. Test the indicator muscle.
5. Record if the muscle is now weak, or strong.
6. Isn't that interesting? Now look at the color blue in the sky. Is the indicator muscle now weak, or is it strong?
7. Discuss and repeat, if necessary.
8. Test many colors. Which seem to weaken and "switch-off"? Which strengthen and switch on?

Karen (not a true name), a third grade teacher, saw immediate changes in her class when she started wearing greens, blues, and purples, and stopped wearing pinks, oranges and reds.

SOUNDS AND MUSIC

Now that we have introduced the idea that certain light rays hitting our energy fields at particular vibrations might upset our energy balance, we can easily study sound, which we already know strikes our eardrums as vibrations.

We have all experienced the importance of music in influencing our emotions. Movie soundtracks may make us feel frightened or nostalgic. Music may make us want to march patriotically or dance with frenzied abandon. Sounds make us feel sleepy or help us to get our work done. Let's test what some common sounds in our environment do to our Energy levels!

SUGGESTED SOUNDS AND MUSIC TO TEST FOR YOURSELVES
1. Running water
2. Rock music

3. Classical music
   a. allegro
   b. adante
4. Kitchen appliances and machines

FOR EXAMPLE:
1. Test an indicator muscle in the clear.
2. Play rock music for thirty seconds.
3. Retest the indicator muscle.
4. Does it test weak or strong? Record findings.

Experiments with a learning technique popularly known as "Superlearning" (as reported by Ostrander and Schroeder in their book of that title) utilizes slow and stately classical music, about 60 beats per minute, to help students learn languages in a relaxed, passive, receptive manner, free from anxiety. We are having similar successes using music in conjunction with our work with learning disabilities at Valley Remedial Group. William, a rock fan, asked to hear that "slow" music again, because it helped him to concentrate. Stan doesn't lose his place when he reads if he listens to soft, slow music in the background. In addition, the therapists show much more patience since we have music. Perhaps this is the most significant development.

FOODS AND OUR ENERGY FIELDS

Perhaps the most suspected culprit in our environment when it comes to Energy blockage is processed food. The health food industry has been active for several decades, and many books and television interviews have bombarded us with the importance of a natural diet and vitamins. Edu-Kinesthetics does not endorse any one diet, and no one but a licensed doctor may prescribe a diet or vitamin supplements. Edu-Kinesthetics does help people decide for themselves which foods give them maximum Energy and which seem to switch them off. Simply select a variety of foods which you normally eat or would like to eat, and place them, one at a time, in your mouth without swallowing. Rinse your mouth with water between foods. Head your paper with three columns, for you will discover that foods can be strengthening, weakening, or neutral. A strengthening food will change a weak muscle to strong, a weakening food will weaken a strong muscle, and a neutral food will have no effect on a muscle. It will remain weak or strong depending upon the food previously eaten. Mary Jane came to class clutching a bag of cookies. She was so relieved that they tested "neutral." She really did not want to give them up.

You might wish to repeat food testing over a period of weeks or months, for results do change as you become more centered and balanced. Assume only that for your present situation, these foods make you respond in this manner. If you should choose to experiment with your food testing findings, eliminate a food, and feel better, perform better, and have more energy, the results would be clear.

The Latissimus Dorsi is the best indicator muscle for food testing; however, any muscle will do.

THE POWER OF WORDS

"There's been a breakdown in communication." These famous last words are all too true. Just attempt to write a book or teach a class, and you will soon find out how easy it is to be ambiguous when using language. When each person's experience is unique to himself, our words may denote the same thing, but have entirely different connotations to all concerned. Words that are relative to something that is not absolute are a good example. How big is big? What is good behavior? How late is really late?

When it comes to learning and performing, there seem to be certain words which switch off Energy. These words connote a negative state or promote failure, even though this does not appear to be the conscious meaning intended. No one likes to be evaluated. When you use words that are judgmental it creates unnecessary stress.

Muscle test these words with your partner. If he tests weak on his indicator muscle, switch to the alternate way to express the same idea. I think you will find it very interesting!

Test Word	Alternate Word or Phrase
can't	not able, unable
try	do, be
forgot	didn't remember
failed	didn't succeed
hope to	will
lost	didn't win
stretch	reach, grow
problem	challenge

NATURAL VS. PLASTIC

Our environment has become increasingly more artificial, synthetic, and man-made, and many of us are so sensitive to a plastic world that it adversely affects our Energy balance. It makes sense to retain the benefits of modern life, but to eliminate those plastics which we do not really need. We are natural and evolved to live in nature. The more we keep in contact with nature, the better we can function.

The list of natural and plastic items is endless, so experiment with items you think are weakening or strengthening. Below are some natural and plastic items we have tested with students:
- wood vs. formica and plastic chairs and tables;
- jewelry, plastic vs. real gems;
- synthetic fibers in clothes vs. cotton, wool, silk and leather;
- artificial light vs. sunlight;
- makeup, synthetic vs. natural ingredients

TELEVISION

Television, and films for that matter, ask us to use our eyes in a two-dimensional, unnatural way. It is unbalancing and certainly aggravates the condition of a child with a tendency for visual problems. Muscle testing television viewing consistently shows its negative influence on one's energy balance. Please test it for yourself. Unless you can justify the negative influence, do not watch television and drastically reduce or eliminate your child's television viewing.

PEOPLE

Perhaps the most important factor in our environment is our contact with the people with whom we live, and encounter in our work and play. Hundreds of books have been written on the subject, and the helping professions proliferate with psychologists, psychiatrists, and counselors for every human interaction.

Edu-Kinesthetics can be used to demonstrate the power of our nonverbal, hidden attitudes when we enter another's Lifespace. Often these attitudes are hidden from our own consciousness, as well as the second person's, and can be quite unintentional. Once determined by muscle testing, thoughtful people can change their behavior to create an environment which strengthens instead of weakens.

The testing is the same as for the other environmental testing, except now we are testing the power of thought! Send someone out of the room, and write down, on separate cards, in any order, a list of four or five attitudes, both positive and negative. For example:
You are beautiful;
You are incapable;
I love you;
I cannot work with you;
I feel rotten today;
I feel good when I'm with you.
Call the person back, and begin the testing. The person who thinks the thought, tests the muscles.

PROCEDURE:
1. Test a strong indicator muscle in the clear.
2. Think thought number 1 for several seconds and repeat the test. Note whether strong, or weak.
3. Repeat with thoughts 2, 3, 4, etc. Note responses.
4. Did weak responses coincide with the negative attitudes?
5. Did strong responses coincide with positive attitudes?
6. Show individual the list, and explain what you did.

We have found that a person doing muscle testing must be reasonably balanced. Often an individual will test weak in a muscle for no other reason than that the testor is weak. Mothers, when testing their children, find weaknesses that do not exist for others. If this is due to the mother's or child's negativity outwardly toward each other, or inwardly toward themselves, whether conscious or unconscious, steps can be taken to correct the situation. One step is to learn to put the mind in a neutral state where no particular response is expected. Just relax and do the test quickly. The chapter on dealing with emotional stress will teach another technique which is very useful in communications.

CHAPTER IV
STRESS AND NEGATIVE THINKING
"He makes me sick to my stomach."
"My stomach is all tied up in knots."
"I hate his/her guts!"

Our casual conversation reflects all too well the true nature of our being. Negative thinking is directed to and is experienced in the stomach. Be it worry, fear, anxiety, unpleasant memories, or poor self-image, these emotions all take up residence there, whether we like it or not. Physically, these emotions can lead to stomach aches, indigestion, ulcers, and possibly to more serious problems as the system degenerates.

Why does "stress" hit us where we "live"? Neurologically we have evolved to respond to stress with a survival instinct. The "fight or flight" response is controlled by the limbic system at the top of the brain stem, but not physically a part of either the right or left brain. The limbic system controls the sympathetic/parasympathetic nerves which, in turn, control the viscera (heart, lungs, liver, intestines, etc.) and all the blood vessels in the body. As we go through life, we operate on "automatic pilot," relying upon stimulus-response habit patterns to eliminate decisions. If we had to think mentally about each action we take, we could never get out of bed in the morning. The body, to survive, learns a computerized program for all situations that it has ever experienced.

Imagine that you are challenged for a fight. Blood rushes to the face, neck, arms and chest to prepare you for a physical confrontation. That is why our faces flush when we are angry. When frightened, the opposite happens, as blood is drawn away from the upper torso to supply Energy for running away. In extreme cases, our faces pale, we get speechless, stutter, or forget everything. A case can be made that fight is a primitive left-brain response, and flight is right-brained; however, the decision is made below the level of consciousness. Both are correct responses to actual danger to the organism, but we do not need these responses in most of our day-to-day, civilized encounters.

REDUCING STRESS

Yoga and meditation are recognized methods for reducing stress, and proponents of these techniques claim that stress-related illnesses can be eliminated and performance of all kinds improved by learning these disciplines. Biofeedback monitoring, as pioneered by Elmer Green, has demonstrated that the yogi, when concentrating or meditating, has conscious control of the activities performed by the limbic system and usually performed only on the subconscious level. By sending blood and Energy to different organs and different parts of the body voluntarily, fakirs perform their "magic" tricks, such as lying upon nails without bleeding. Biofeedback can provide the same abilities to modern man by allowing him to "know" by feedback that he has produced a voluntary change in his system. Edu-Kinesthetics provides a similar type of feedback, without the electronic equipment.

In the 1930's Dr. Bennett, a chiropractor, discovered that there were locations on the head, which, if held, seemed to influence blood supply to certain organs. In the 1960's, Dr. George Goodheart, the father of Applied Kinesiology, found that he could strengthen a weak muscle by stimulating the appropriate "Bennett reflex." The "weak" muscle indicates that the blood supply of the body is out of balance, with excessive amounts going to areas involved in the "fight or flight" response and, simultaneously, being drawn from other areas. Holding the appropriate "Bennett reflex" restored the blood flow to "normal" and this was indicated by the strong, locked muscle.

When the survival instinct is threatened, certainly no learning can take place, nor can one perform well, whatever his chosen profession. Yet parents, teachers, employers, and "the system" place us continually "under fire." Emotional stress is often the primary factor in muscle imbalances. No muscle balancing will take place until the emotional stress is relieved. When the individual is relaxed and secure within himself at the visceral level, and is no longer threatened, his self-concept will accept instruction, correction, and opportunities for growth and change.

Edu-Kinesthetics uses the pectoralis major clavicular muscle to test for emotional stress. (Refer to Chapter II.) If it tests weak on a routine muscle test, it is safe to assume that there is stress involved. The person may volunteer this information, but there is no need to suggest it and further aggravate the situation. Instead, lightly hold the Frontal Eminences on the forehead of the individual as indicated in Figure 1. Hold just tight enough to gently pull the skin taut and feel for the slightest pulsations beneath the skin under each hand. John Thie states that this pulse is not related to heartbeat, but is probably the primitive pulsation of the microscopic capillary bed in the skin. After the pulse has been felt on both sides, hold until they are equalized. This will take from about twenty seconds to up to ten minutes, depending upon the nature of the stress.

Note the changes in the individual. If beforehand he was unable to read or talk, he now can concentrate and speak with a normal tone of voice. He is more able to mentally deal with stress, and rationally execute a plan of action which may accomplish a solution to the problem. A similar result to the meditation of the yogi has been accomplished, and the feedback is in the retest of the pectoralis major clavicular muscle. It can now be locked, indicating that emotional balance has been restored. The problem may still exist, but his emotional response to it is now different, and the individual can more easily go about dealing with it without his body treating it like there is a threat to his survival.

Edu-Kinesthetics suggests many preventative and therapeutic applications of this technique for release of emotional stress. They combine the meditative and feedback aspects with holding the Frontal Eminences. You can do these exercises with a partner, or alone by yourself if no partner is available.

PROCEDURE FOR EMOTIONAL STRESS RELEASE:
1. Select either the strong pectoralis major clavicular or supraspinatus muscle.
2. Ask the subject to think about a "negative" thought.
3. Retest the muscle. It will be weak.
4. Hold the Frontal Eminences as indicated above.

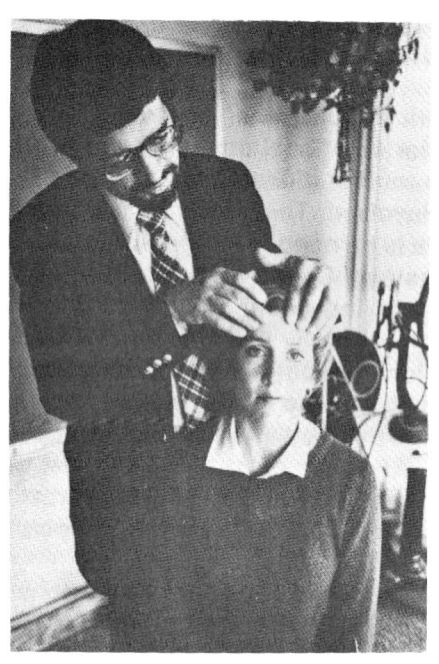

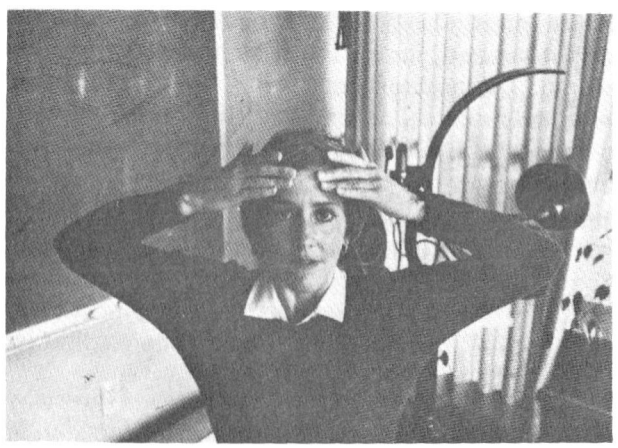

1 Position of the hands when holding the Frontal Eminences on the forehead to reduce emotional stress.

5. Retest the muscle. It will be strong.
6. Direct the subject to think about the "negative" thought again.
7. Test the muscle. It should remain strong!

Suggested applications, all to be done while holding Frontal Eminences:

1. *Role playing:*
   Play a movie in your mind of a past negative experience until you test strong.
2. *Anticipating stresses:*
   Tests, oral reading or interviews can be rehearsed until you test strong.
3. *Changing reactions to selected persons:*
   Think of the person's name or face until you test strong.
4. *Changing reactions to negative factors in the environment:*
   Imagine the negative factor, using as many different sensory modes as possible, until you test strong.

Everyone seems to have a unique reason for "switching off" be it mental, physical, spiritual, or emotional. If the reason is related to self-concept, and one has an overactive "fight or flight" mechanism, creative applications of the technique of holding the Frontal Eminences can be the most beneficial part of Edu-Kinesthetics.

CHAPTER V
CROSS-MOTOR PATTERNING

DYSLEXIA AND LEARNING DISABILITIES

I first realized that cross-motor patterning would help with learning disabilities shortly after taking a "Touch for Health" course from Dick Harnack. Dick emphasized "cross-crawling" and I was the volunteer. The experience of strengthening and weakening through bilateral and homolateral movements intrigued me profoundly, and I decided to include it in my therapy. The first student I taught to cross-crawl was Judy, a fifteen-year-old dyslexic who was having particular difficulty that day with a fourth grade reading book. After she cross-crawled, the phone rang and my back was to her as she began to read again, aloud. To my amazement, I heard a voice reading which sounded completely different with perfect phrasing, word recognition, and comprehension. It was a different Judy, relaxed, poised, and confident. The cross-crawling had balanced her and altered her performance level. Great! But why did she need to be balanced? And what does balancing do for the dyslexic? These questions led to intensive research and investigation at our offices.

Now, almost a year later, the answers are both simple and revolutionary, and my questions are answered. Diagnosis, counseling, and therapy are a joyful adventure. Teaching and learning need never be drudgery again. Dyslexics try too hard. Afraid they will fail, or pushed to succeed, they concentrate too intensely, switching off all peripheral information as they zero in on one thing. Dyslexics are simply experts at blocking

Energy. From the moment of birth, they have been compensating for a lowered energy level with inefficient information processing. Easy learning requires integration of right-brain and left-brain functioning so that the whole is always perceived as more than the sum of its parts. The left brain must be conscious of language and comprehension, and the right brain must deal with symbols and the code. This is done automatically and subconsiously.

Muscle balancing allows dyslexics to read and write efficiently for the first time, keeping all information processing systems on and functioning at all times. Through misinterpretation of the role of handedness and dominance in reading, treatment of dyslexia has been, historically, left-brain training emphasizing drills in sequencing, order, and phonetics. The dyslexic is taught to match speech sounds to written symbols. The complexity of the English language makes it a hopeless task for most true dyslexics, and only makes them switch off more.

Pioneers in dyslexia, such as Orton and Delacato, and most other educators, have overlooked the role of the right brain in learning and information processing. The right brain is intuitive, spontaneous, rhythmic and expressive. It opens the body to a total awareness. When the right brain is "switched-on," Energy flows through the whole body, muscles are balanced, and the universe is perceived as a "gestalt" or whole. The details are less important than the perception of meaning. This is how language is learned by children. There is no "trying" or "effort" to synthesize parts to make the whole. This is done by the child himself, naturally, as he grows and gains confidence in self-expression. The dyslexic, whether through birth trauma, congenital birth defect, emotional stress, or hyperactivity, does not integrate right brain and left brain automatically when dealing with symbols. Some can memorize words up to a certain level, but can neither write nor spell them. Others can read and spell by sound synthesis, but cannot recognize nor visualize words as a whole.

Training the dyslexic to perform left-brain skills when he is unbalanced and "blocking" only compounds the problem. With his right brain "switched off," he has poor use of his natural creative, visualizing skills, and he will not be able to see things as "wholes," as he tries too hard to analyze and break things down into tiny bits of data. He cannot learn to use recognition, insight, and communicate beyond the literal level. He doesn't use imagination or visualization. When balanced with a heightened Energy level, the dyslexic is more able to relax and experience integration of the hemispheres when dealing with symbols. He learns that "trying" only blocks Energy. He realizes that he knows far more than he thought, and that he could not retrieve it through self-caused stress and blockage. He learns that reading is fun and easy when the body's energies are flowing and in balance.

DON, A DYSLEXIC
    Don is twenty-nine and could hardly read at the third grade level when he came to me, pointing to one word at a time. He had spent a fortune going from one expert to another and from clinic to clinic. He felt they were interested in studying him, but could not help him. He was told that he could not visualize and would never read. Don's posture was poor, with rounded shoulders and shortened neck from years of not turning his head. He was bilaterally weak in the supraspinatus, pectoralis major clavicular, and latissimus dorsi muscles, a pattern typical of ninety percent of my clientele. Don complained of tightness in his chest when under stress, and reading and writing caused shortness of breath and stiffness in the right side of his body, and reading was obviously hard physical work for him. Cross-crawling helped Don immediately, and he became more relaxed and volunteered that his back felt good for the first time in years!
    Don, after six months of training, reads independently at the sixth grade level. He reads with fluency and ease. He is aware of his body and stays balanced through self regulation. He no longer requires a teacher for emotional support and reinforcement. He still may have a lot to learn about reading and writing, and these will improve with time and effort. He knows he is no longer dyslexic; that is the important thing for right now.

WHAT IS CROSS-MOTOR PATTERNING OR CROSS-CRAWLING?
    Cross-motor patterning is any rhythmic, balanced movement which requires the individual to dynamically relate the right side of his body to the left side of his body, while at the same time being aware of the top half of his body and the lower half. (See Figure 1)

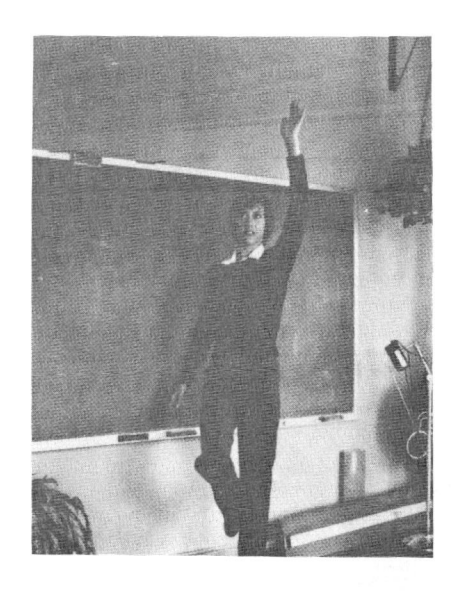

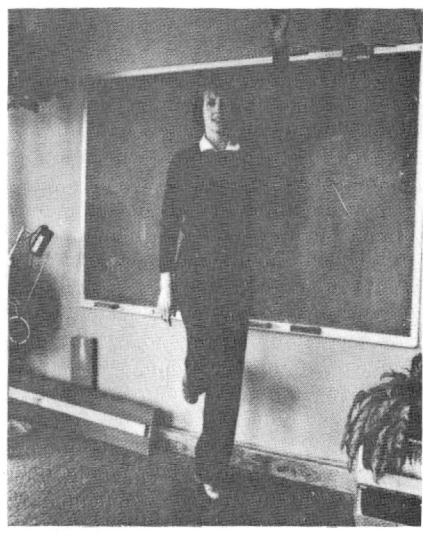

Fig. 1 Cross motor patterning is any rhythmic, balanced movement which requires the individual to dynamically relate the right side of his body to the left side of his body, while, at the same time, being aware of the top half of his body and the lower half.

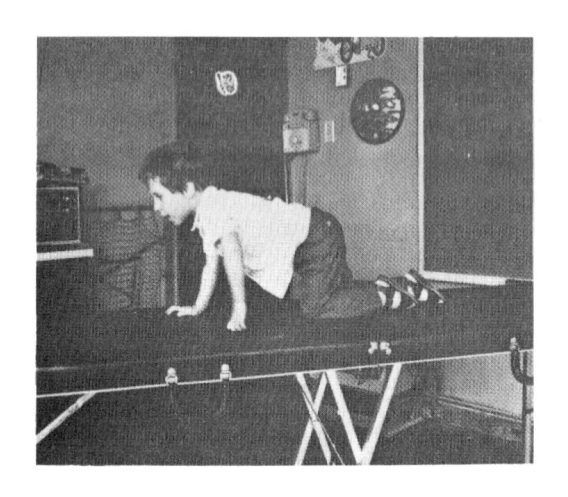

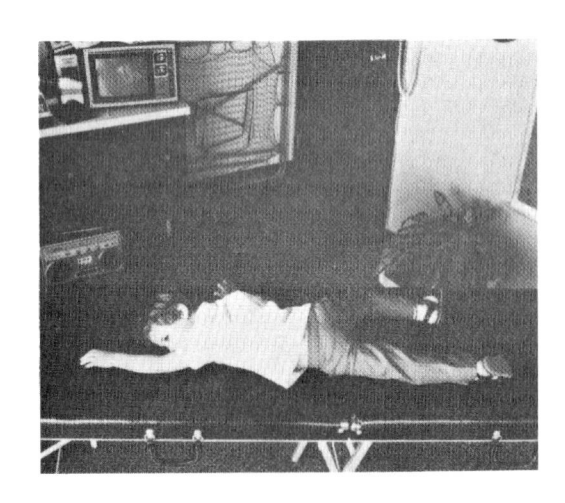

Fig. 2 Actual creeping and crawling. The head turns in the direction of the forward arm.

Cross-crawling requires precise switching on and off of muscles by the brain at exactly the right time, and requires feedback and feedforward from and to the muscles to maintain the exercise. This highly intricate bilateral integration is learned by the infant during the creeping and crawling stages before walking. It is the same type of cooperation of the cerebral hemispheres that is required for reading and writing. It seems that most dyslexics have not internalized cross-motor patterning, and therefore have difficulty when returning to it. It is easy to skip this developmental stage in childhood and function quite normally. Most activities do not require synchronized brain patterns. But the rewards seem endless once this developmental stage has been learned. (See figure 2.)

WHO NEEDS CROSS-CRAWLING?

Cross-crawling is a normal motor activity and is good for everyone. It is fun and relaxing. You can do it any time you are tense, nervous, or tired, at home, at school, or at the office.

If your student reports that he has trouble reading, or hates to do so, he probably will have trouble cross-crawling. If he is weak on any of our indicator muscles, especially the Supraspinatus, he may be a candidate for cross-crawling as well.

SUGGESTED PROCEDURES
1. Test the indicator muscles. Identify weaknesses, if any.
2. Demonstrate the cross-crawl exercise and observe whether the individual performs it in a bilateral (opposite arm and leg) or homolateral (same arm and leg) pattern.
3. If a homolateral pattern is used, demonstrate the cross-crawl again, and instruct him to watch you lift one arm and the opposite leg at one time as if you were crawling on your hands and knees on the floor. Tell him to feel this as he thinks about his own body.
4. If this is unsuccessful, actual crawling or patterning of the individual while lying on his back may be required. (See figure 3.)

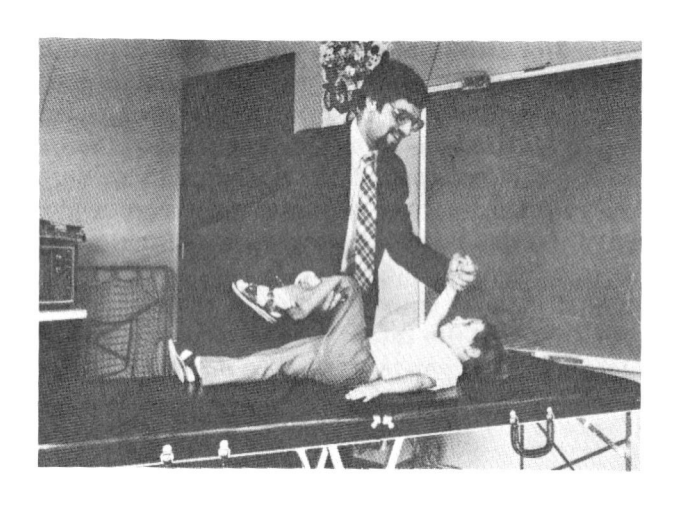

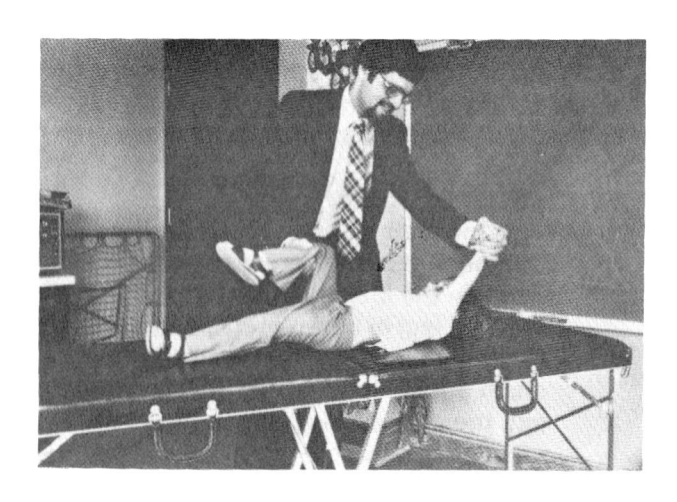

Fig. 3 Patterning of the individual while lying on his back is the most therapeutic method.

5. When cross-crawling is accomplished by one of the above methods, retest the indicator muscles. If the individual is strengthened, then he will be helped to understand that cross-crawling is a developmental task which is necessary for normal intellectual functioning.
6. Ask the individual to use a homolateral crawl. Test an indicator muscle. If weakened, your subject experiences how easily he can be "switched-off."
7. Teach how to "switch on." Besides cross-crawling physically in one of the illustrated patterns, it must be emphasized that this is a mental act involving voluntary mental processes which keep Energy flowing properly.
    a) Imagine that you are cross-crawling. Do you test strong, or weak?
    b) Imagine that you are homolateral crawling. Do you test strong, or weak?
    c) Visualize a crossed figure, an X. Do you test strong, or weak?
    d) Visualize two parallel lines, a number 11. Do you test strong, or weak?

TEACHING AND LEARNING SUGGESTIONS

Cross-crawling is most easily taught with people standing in place or marching around the room. Arms and legs should be lifted vigorously and lightness on the feet is necessary (see Chapter six). Cross-crawling in this manner is convenient, manageable for the teacher, and fun for the group. Muscle testing has proven that this approach is sufficient to balance most cases for improved learning ability. When difficulty persists for an individual in grasping cross-crawling, your understanding of the process as experienced by the individual will help him to master it in due time.

Developmentally, one who is having difficulty cross-crawling is more comfortable at the homolateral stage where the arm and leg on the same side move together as a reflex. This is the stage when the newborn infant will lie on his back and move his limbs simultaneously. It is also the stage when the infant crawls on his tummy with his head on the floor so that only one eye can see at one time. If an individual tests "strong" after a homolateral crawl and "weak" after a cross-crawl, he is certainly at this stage neurologically.

Many homolateral crawlers have learned to inhibit or switch off one eye. Cross-crawling is readily accomplished, as if by magic, as soon as both eyes are switched on (See Chapter seven)! When the right-brain eye is switched-on, the individual can both think and feel movement at the same time. Cross-crawling must be practiced until it gets totally automatic and requires minimal analysis. Twenty-five repetitions, three or four times per day is sufficient.

For stubborn cases it is effective to require the switched-on individual to crawl in a homolateral style only, reminding him to think about what he is doing. The repeated analysis of his actions, such as, "right arm and leg up, left arm and leg up, etc.," will soon become tiring and will make cross-crawling more attractive. This is an extinction conditioning process, and usually is completed in only a few days. When retested, whether after one month, six months, or after one year, cross-crawling will be strengthening, indicating hemispheric integration and total awareness without stress.

The homolateral crawler is "switched off." Not needing to think analytically to experience this movement, he tests stronger as he repeats a reflex action learned in infancy. When required to think about cross-crawling, however, he must switch off his right brain as he focuses the left brain on the more advanced task. Whenever analytical thought processes cause "stress," one must switch off the part of the brain which feels movement, and muscles test weak. In order to grow from the homolateral stage to the cross-crawl stage, one needs to reverse the thought processes which cause the switching off. One needs to think analytically to crawl homolaterally instead of relying on reflex, and one needs to become automatic and stay switched on while cross-crawling. E-K methods accomplish this development.

Margaret, an adult in her thirties, was a homolateral crawler. She would test "strong" after jumping jacks or marching in place, raising the arm and leg on the same side of her body. She would test "weak" when asked to perform a cross-motor patterned activity.

Observation of her eye movements suggested that homolateral crawling required no analytical thought as she pointed her eyes to the left, activating her right brain (See Chapter seven). She could do these simply by reflex action. When asked to cross-crawl, she appeared confused and hesitant, looking to the right, activating the left brain and freezing her body stiffly. Cross-crawling required her constant concentration to monitor her body movements.

Explaining what was happening, I suggested doing the opposite with her eyes, and required more analysis of the homolateral crawl as she looked right. I suggested looking to the left, when cross-crawling, visualizing and feeling the movements as she practiced them. She tested strong immediately when cross-crawling this way and soon overcame her hesitancy about integrated learning activities.

EVAULATION OF RESULTS
1. Do reading and writing spontaneously improve?
2. Does cross-crawling become automatic, no demonstrations required?
3. Does testing the indicator muscle, without cross-crawling immediately beforehand, find the muscle strong and locked? Neurological patterns are strengthened and internal coordination develops and new beneficial, balanced habits are formed.

(See Figures 4, 5, and 6 for alternative cross-crawl patterns which may be enjoyed using a musical accompaniment.)

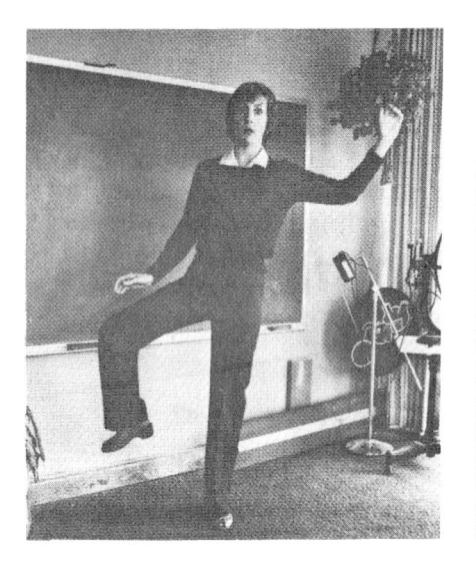

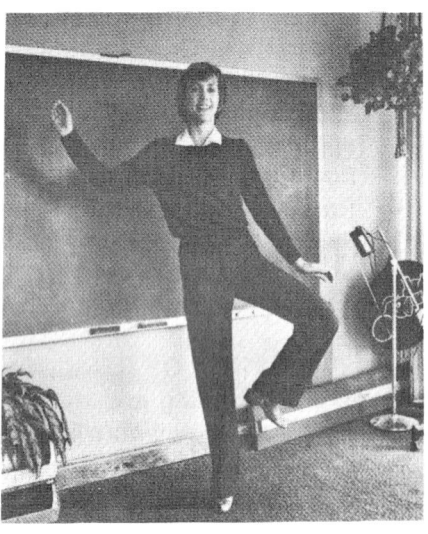

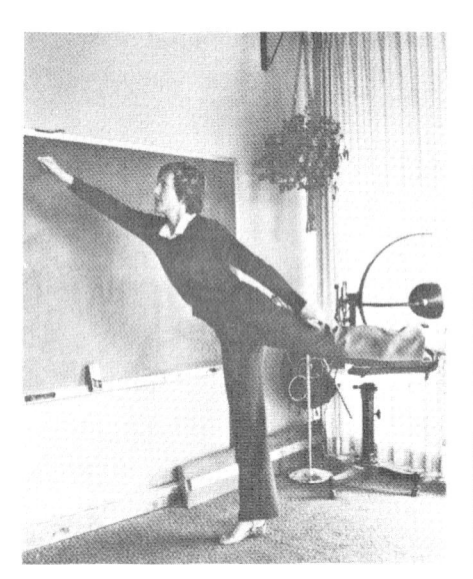

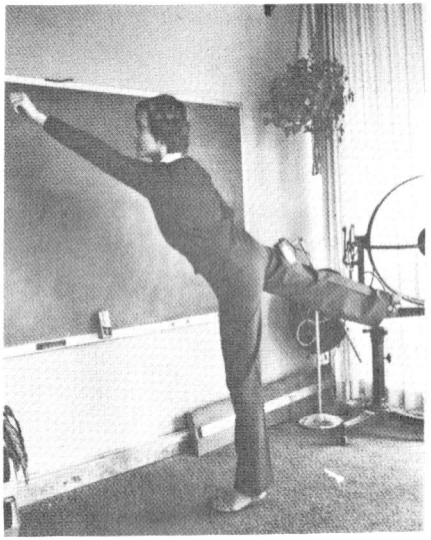

Fig. 4 Two cross-motor patterns which can be enjoyed using musical accompaniment.

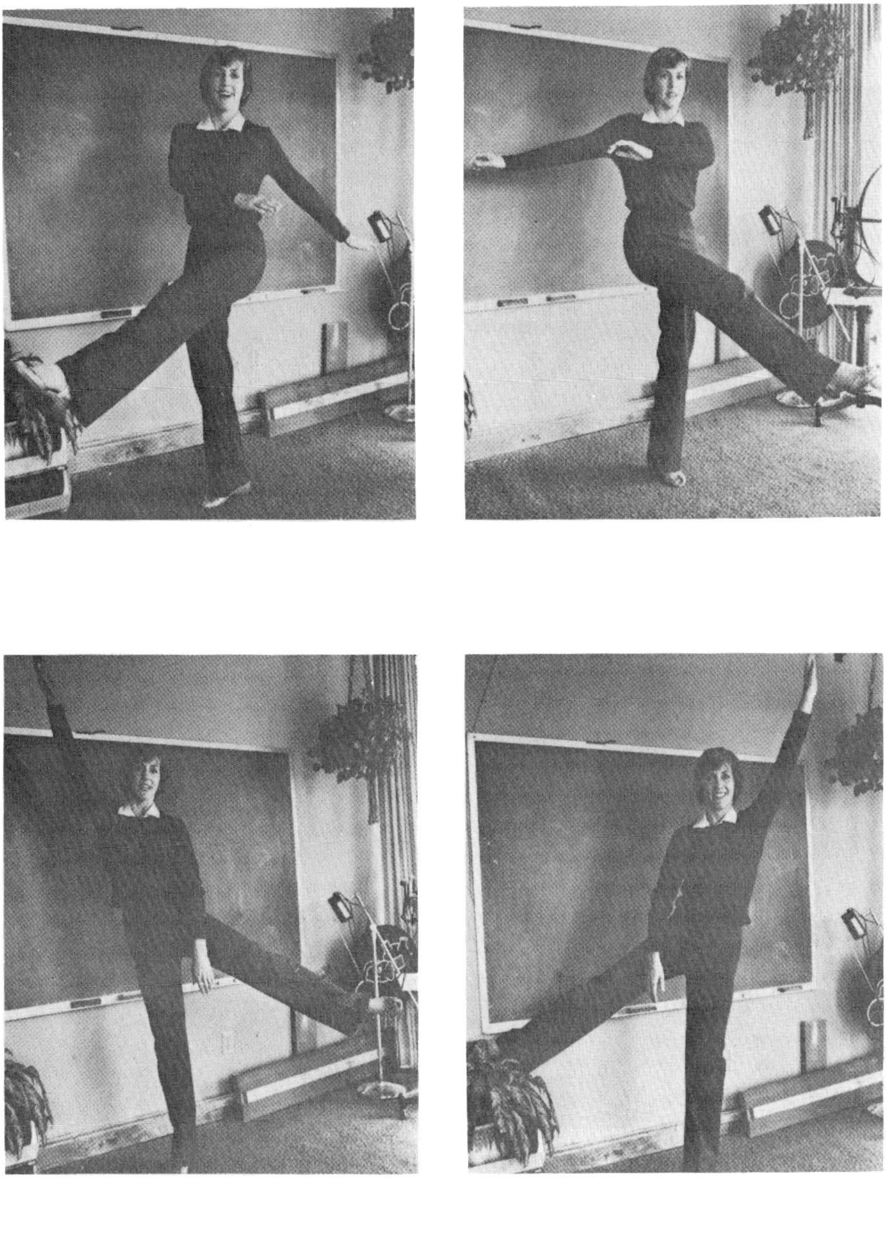

Fig. 5 Two cross-motor patterns which can be enjoyed using musical accompaniment.

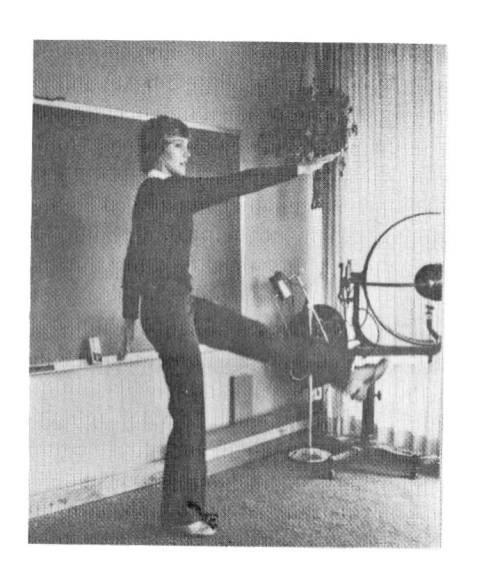

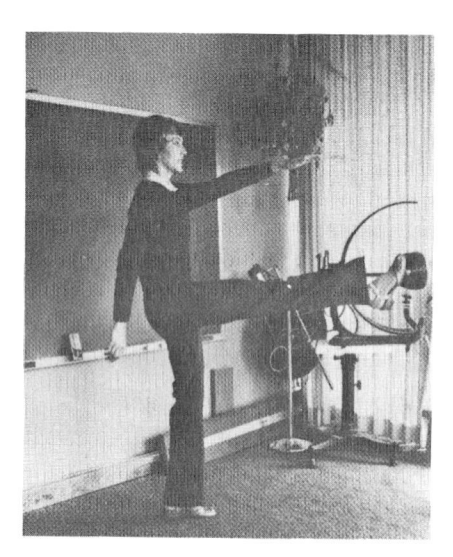

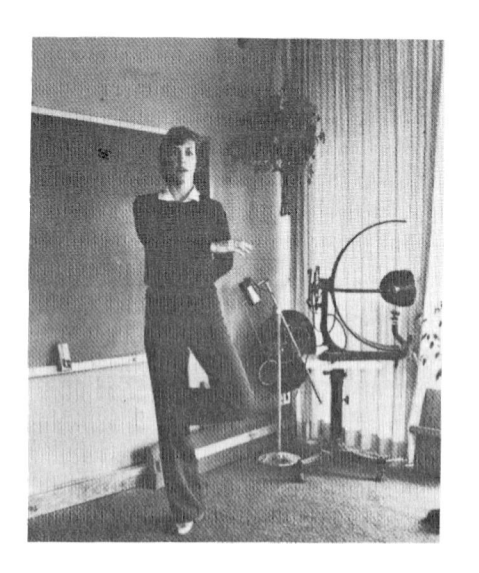

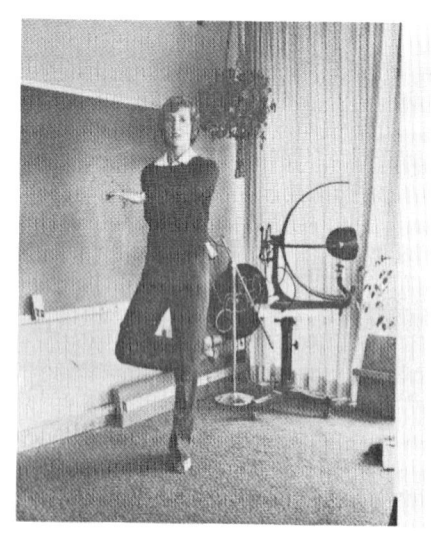

Fig. 6 Two cross-motor patterns which can be enjoyed using musical accompaniment.

CHAPTER VI
POSTURE FROM WITHIN

"How long will I stay balanced?" This is the question heard most often by our educational therapists. It is easy enough to criticize poor posture and correct irregularities with E-K techniques, but we can really only help people improve if we teach them to stay balanced, use muscles properly, and maintain good posture.

When we look at young children, playing, running, and laughing, with beautiful erect bodies, we wonder what happens to create the postural deviations we see in the adult population. Accidents, illnesses, and stress are the culprits! When people recover from some traumatic life experience, muscles remember and are "switched-off." One compensates for weak muscles or pain by neglecting certain movements and overusing others. The new movements soon become habitual. The resulting "bad" posture is a picture of imbalance.

Theoretically, when the body of an individual is balanced, he has a chance to regain the perfect posture of his youth. The years of bad habits and a poor self-image will soon return the body to its customary condition, however, unless posture and movement reeducation is introduced as part of a caring counseling program.

A significant part of our therapy involves posture and movement reeducation or "Edu-Kinesthetics." The success of our program depends upon the student relearning to use his body correctly and elevating his self-image. The academics, although necessary, are really the least important part of the program.

I first became involved with posture education through my own personal back and shoulder problems. I have invested hundreds of hours in interventions to improve my posture such as structural integration (Rolfing), Structural Patterning, self-hypnosis, Chiropractic treatment, orthotic devices, yoga, etc. All have helped somewhat, but none brought relief from the pain or corrected the posture to my satisfaction. From each I learned what to do and what not to do as well. I am now often complimented on my posture, and it was finally achieved through understanding and controlling Energy, and by eliminating "trying" so hard as I had always done.

THE NECK IS CRITICAL

In order to move about in good posture, stand erect, think, express oneself fluently, and learn, the neck must be free to conduct Energy. The importance of the neck cannot be overemphasized. If the neck is open, relaxed, and loose, the body and mind can work together. When the neck is closed and tight, it actually becomes a valve to shut off Energy and performance is crippled. When students learn the importance of the neck, through muscle testing, they are better able to maintain awareness of their bodies and take control of their own lives.

BALANCE DIMENSIONS

Balance has many dimensions. We usually think of balance in terms of side-to-side or left-to-right as in balancing the "scales of justice" or balancing on a tightrope. Energy balancing certainly includes bilateral integration of the two sides of the body, but there are other dimensions of equal or greater importance. One is front-to-back, back-to-front balance, and the other is up-and-down, down-and-up equilibrium. The former is seriously neglected in our culture and is the cause of many back ills. The latter is yang-yin, gravity-anti-gravity Energy flow and the most important part of our work. Without this dimension, none of the other balancing will hold and posture may deteriorate.

Ask the child who has just fallen down about gravity, and he will tell you that it hurts! Gravity is a constant which holds our world together. We can depend upon it, and we must continually compensate for its pull. It draws our Energy down, and if we let it control us, it can make us feel heavy. If we let gravity's pull sap our bodies, we feel weak, tired, and slumped as if we were carrying the burden of the world on our shoulders.

To equalize the pull of gravity, we have a Life Force which flows through us and all living things. Just as it lifts birds to flight and makes trees grow straight and tall, it can make our movement in space beautiful, effortless, and free. When we feel this Force within us and let it flow through our neck and shoulders, we move gracefully and our muscles seem to know what to do without conscious control. Edu-Kinesthetics teaches people how to move in space. When we know how to move, posture takes care of itself.

REPROGRAMMING ENERGY FLOW

The following sequence of muscle tests can be adapted to one's own needs, whether classroom or private instruction. Examination of the tasks and challenges we make to the Energy flow will give you some insight as to the process which must be experienced to change posture. We use the Supraspinatus because it measures best the fatigue involved in learning disabilities. Any indicator muscle will give the same results. (See Figure 1.)

1. Test a strong indicator muscle in the clear.
2. Ask your student to stand up straight and tall. Test the indicator muscle. Response: Invariably this request blocks energy, because people "try too hard" and assume an unnatural posture.
3. If his muscle is weak, strengthen him by running your open hand up the central line of the body from groin to upper lip several times. (It is not necessary to touch.)
    Test the muscle.
    Response: Strong.
4. Ask him how he feels. There should be a difference. (Lighter and relaxed when strong; heavier and tense or anxious when weak.)
5. If necessary, weaken him by running your open hand down the central line of the body so the student can experience and verbalize how he feels each way. Strengthen him again.
6. Weaken his body again. Now tell the student to feel the Energy returning up in his imagination.
    Test the muscle again.
    Response: Strong.

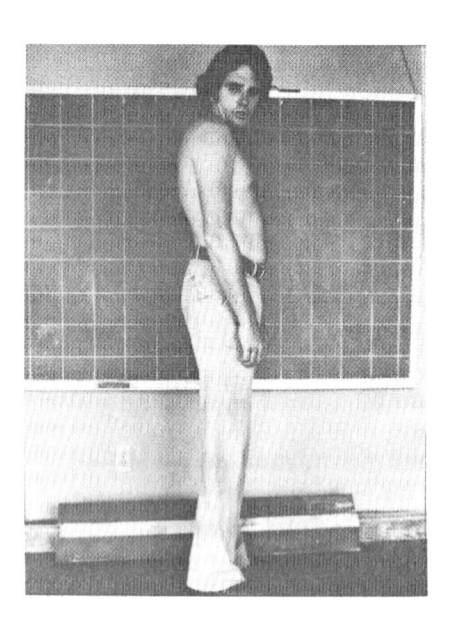

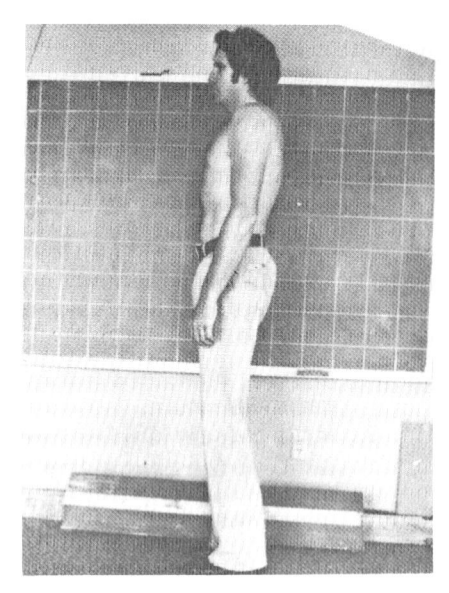

Fig. 1 Postural deviations become readily apparent when studied against a grid or imaginary straight line.

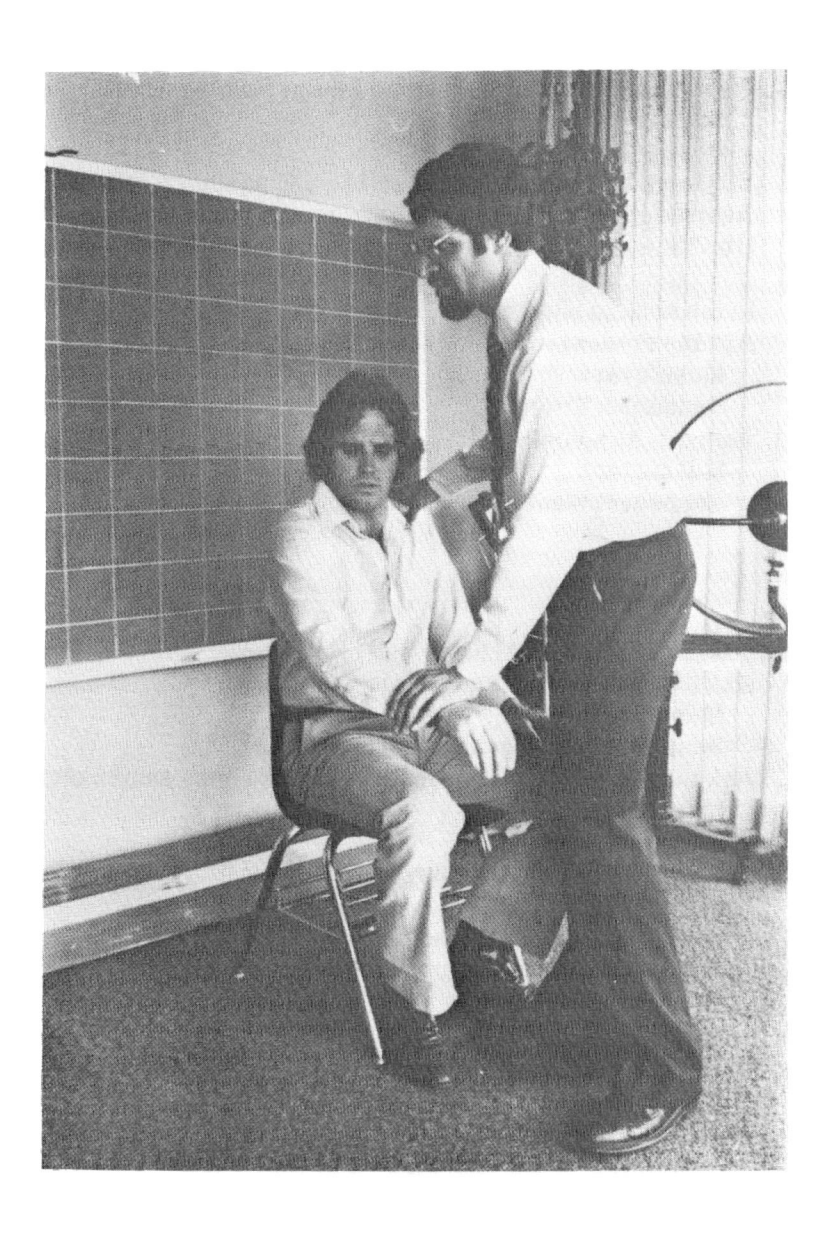

Fig. 2 The act of sitting can change the energy flow through the neck from positive, to negative.

7. Now tell the student to imagine Energy flowing down.
   Muscle test.
   Response: Weak.
8. Tell the student to make himself strong again.
9. Ask the student to concentrate on his neck. Weaken it. How does it feel? Strengthen it. How does it feel? Introduce the image of a valve or a switch that goes on and off in the neck to allow Energy to flow up.
10. Ask the student to turn on the switch.
    Muscle test.
    Response: Strong.
11. Turn off the switch.
    Muscle test.
    Response: Weak.

MOVEMENT RE-EDUCATION   See Figure 2
1. Ask the student to sit down into a chair.
   Muscle test.
   Response: Weak or strong? If weak . . .
2. Ask the student to sit down again with his neck switch on.
   Muscle test.
   Response: Strong.
3. Ask the student to stand up from the chair.
   Muscle test.
   Response: Weak or strong? If weak . . .
4. Ask the student to stand up with his neck switch on.
   Muscle test.
   Response: Strong.
5. Sitting in a desk, ask the student to read a few lines silently.
   Muscle test.
   Response: Weak or strong? If weak . . .
6. Ask the student to read with his neck switch on.
   Muscle test.
   Response: Strong.
7. Ask the student to write several lines on a paper.
   (See Figure 3)
   Muscle test.
   Response: Weak or strong? If weak . . .

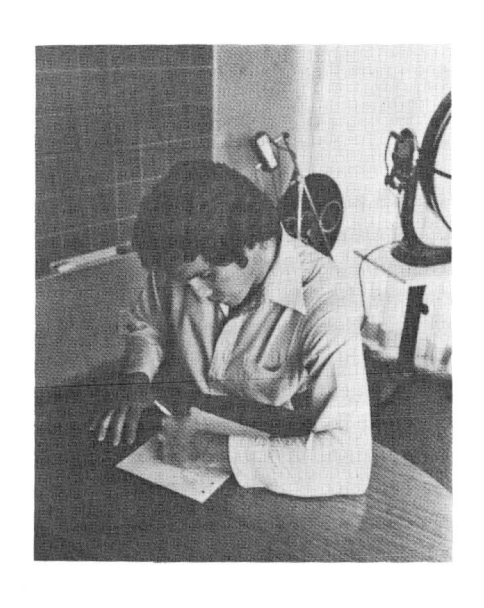

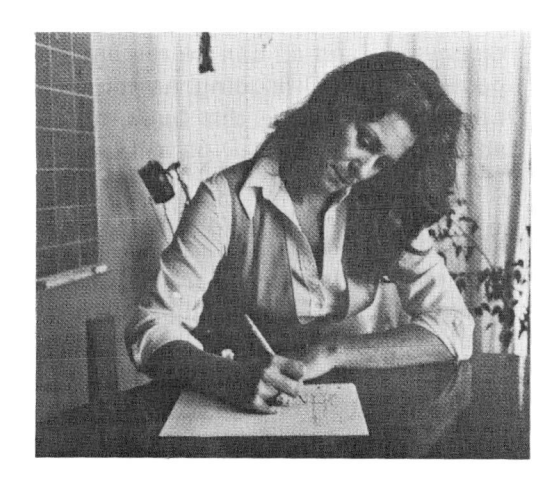

Fig. 3 The act of writing can change the energy flow through the neck from positive, to negative.

8. Ask the student to find a posture where the neck switch stays on and write.
   Muscle test.
   Response: Strong.

POSTURAL ANALYSIS

The above can be done for all activities. Of particular importance are walking, running, singing, eating, speaking and the sports activities of the individual. Practice over a period of time will reinforce the positive habits. In helping students, observe their posture to see how their necks get closed. If they bend the neck forward, balance this movement with a relaxed stretch backward and use the muscle test to show how this opens the valve for Energy flow. If they hold their breath to lock the neck, teach them how to breathe Energy into the open neck. Reinforce with muscle testing. If they stiffen muscles on one side of the body, or use only one eye to read or write, show them how this is affecting the flow of Energy to the neck. Let them discover, with your guidance, what they must do for themselves to achieve openness and balance. If the tongue seems to be involved, show how the tongue's placement will weaken balance, if the tongue is right, left, or thrusted forward, and how balance is strengthened by pressing the tongue up against the palate.

Other methods to keep Energy high and flowing have been discovered and all can be remembered and used to keep the positive flow of life going. As you try these techniques, and the others presented in this book, note which work best for you and your students and you will have the key to a "switched on" posture.

VISUALIZING

In order to internalize good posture, you must see uplifting, energizing, and joyful things around you and within your mind. Your smile or the smile of another will balance you. See a happy face in your mind and you will grow in height. See a sad face and you switch off, slouch and weaken.

Visualize a tree, a soaring bird, or a mountain peak and test your strength.

What symbols connote strength to you? A church steeple, a lucky number, a photograph of someone special. Use muscle testing to identify what makes you feel tall.

FEELING

Even better than seeing it, is feeling it. Become the tree, sinking roots deep and reaching higher and straighter as life's Energy circulates. Feel how light and free you are as you move without apparent effort. Experience the feeling of love one human being has for another. A love that makes no demands or asks for nothing in return. The love of a mother for her child or a child for his pet. When the Energy of unconditional love flows, there is no Energy blockage.

BEING

Feel how good it is right now. Forget the future problems and past mistakes, and experience the present. All time, past, present and future is now, and if you stay balanced for enough "nows" everything will take care of itself. It always has, and it always will.

ENJOYING

"Laughter is the best medicine," we have often said. It is good to take ourselves less seriously, to see the humor in our mistakes and follies, and even in our triumphs. To feel the joy of living, loving and being alive is the key to good posture.

CHAPTER VII
LATERAL DOMINANCE

HANDEDNESS AND EYEDNESS

Tracey, age 13, hates to read and write. She has trouble pronouncing longer words, such as "patriotism," when she reads, and gets easily embarrassed. When she writes, she cannot seem to include all of the words, and she even forgets what she wants to write. She is an excellent conversationalist, however, and remembers everything she hears. She loves to draw, paint, and she writes her own songs.

Mark, age 15, reads fluently and never had poor grades until he got to Jr. High School. He is quiet and shy, reluctant to talk, and his posture appears tense and slumped forward. He enjoys mathematics, but he is frustrated with most other school subjects now, due to poor reading comprehension.

Edu-Kinesthetics studies lateral dominance to help understand a person's strengths and weaknesses. Ideally, we are born with two hands, two eyes, two ears, and even two brains. For a given task, only one hand, eye, ear, and brain can lead and be dominant; the other must follow.

The right brain controls the left side of the body, and the left brain controls the right side of the body. The nerves or wires to the muscles and sense organs go directly across the body from the controlling brain. When one side of the brain works, the other relaxes or performs tasks requiring no conscious control.

Tracey's dominance pattern was determined by E-K techniques to be:

Right-brained and Right-handed
   and Left-eyed
   and Right-eared
Mark's dominance pattern was determined to be:
Left-brained and Right-handed
   and Right-eyed
   and Left-eared
The most efficient dominance pattern finds completely consistent sidedness. The right-brained individual will use the left hand, left eye, and left ear, and the left-brained individual will use the right hand, right eye, and right ear.

When there is consistency and complete sidedness, the two brains easily harmonize and cooperate, staying switched-on for bilateral integration. When the pattern is inconsistent, and sidedness is mixed, the two brains get confused about when to work and what to do. Energy is drained from the system, and switching off takes place.

Reading, writing, and spelling are uniquely left-brained tasks, and the ideal learner of these skills has the following pattern of dominance:
Left-brained and Right-handed
   and Right-eyed
   and Right-eared
Such a person can consciously think about the language one is decoding and encoding as one reads and writes, directing his hand, eye, and ear to the significant details as he hears the story in his mind. While his left brain is involved in analyzing the facts, his right brain attends to the subconscious processes of word recognition, writing movement, and listening to the rhythm and flow of the words and phrases, organizing the parts into a whole.

The Right-brained learner, or the learner with mixed sidedness does not read and write as easily. He must learn to stay balanced and switched-on by maximizing integration and minimizing periods of confusion and switching off. This book is written to make such integration possible.

The majority of people (believed to be about seventy-five to eighty percent of the population) are right-handed and right-eyed. This means that the left brain is apparently in control and few learning problems exist for this group. Undoubtedly many of this group are actually right-brained, and there is no guarantee that they are living up to their fullest learning potential.

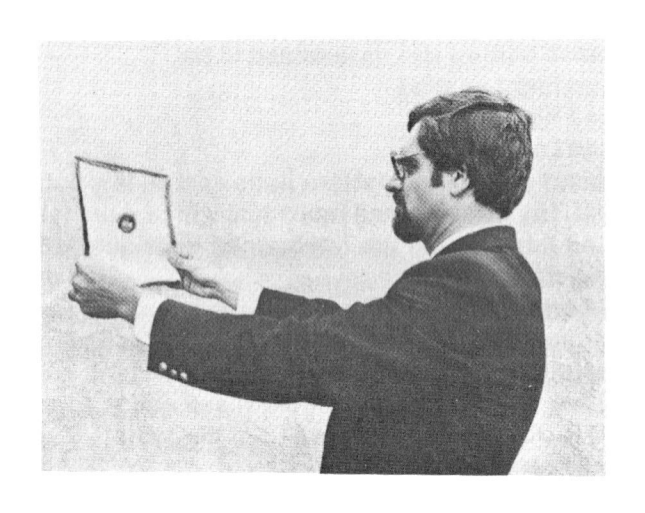

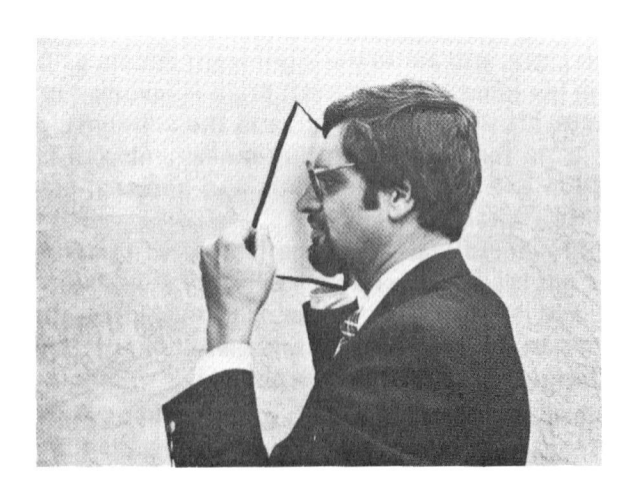

Fig. 1 Test for the determination of one's dominant eye.

The fundamental skills are learned more easily by this group however, and, provided adequate educational opportunities, they appear at remedial reading clinics in small numbers.

About ten percent of the population are left-handed and left-eyed and are thus apparently right-brain dominant. It is difficult to generalize about "lefties" because there are many ways to compensate neurologically. After a period of confusion, which is often traumatic, these people can learn to adjust to a right-handed world of scissors, can openers, ringed notebooks, and school desks. Reading, writing, and spelling were also invented for a right-handed world, and about ten percent of learning disabled children are "lefties."

Another twelve percent of the population are crossed dominant or mixed dominant. Most are right-handed and left-eyed and don't know it. Perhaps they should have been left-handed, but were conditioned otherwise by well-intentioned parents and teachers. Some are left-handed and right-eyed and some are ambidextrous, equally adept with either hand, but with no consistent dominance. Collectively, this group comprises the majority of dyslexics and well over fifty percent of those classified as learning disabled.

Most people have not the slightest notion of their dominant eye or how to test for it. (See Figure 1.)

TEST FOR THE DETERMINATION OF THE DOMINANT EYE

1. Tear a hole in a card or piece of paper and hold it up at arm's length with both hands, so that you focus upon a fixed object, perhaps a coin on the floor or an X on the board.
2. With both eyes open and apparently looking through the hole, move the card up toward the face, keeping the object in sight.
3. This will reveal which eye was actually used to line up the card and the target. Was it the right eye, or left?
4. An enjoyable game is to cover the dominant eye while a child thinks he is looking through the hole with both eyes, making the target disappear. Children are amazed and think it is magic!

BRAINEDNESS AND EYE MOVEMENTS

Studies of the use of the eyes during thought processes suggest that right and left-brained people exist in equal numbers, no matter which hand and eye are apparently dominant.

In Edu-Kinesthetics, the concept of brainedness takes precedence over handedness and eyedness. Those right-handed, right-eyed people who feel frustrated and inhibited in learning may be right-brains without knowing it, although appearing to be left-brained.

The subtle relationship of the eyes to the mind has long been a part of our conventional and folk wisdom. We are "shifty-eyed" or fail to see "eye-to-eye." We are "beady-eyed," or "all eyes," or we don't "see" when something is difficult to understand.

The necessity to use one's eyes to read and write seems obvious, and the ability to move the eyes across the page and back seems so ordinary a task that it is taken for granted. The relationship of this skill to thinking has seldom been considered. It is just a mechanical action that is learned like walking or eating!

Recently, it has been demonstrated that eyes need not "see" to move. The act of thinking, itself, produces CLEMS, "conjugate lateral eye movements" to the left or to the right. When the cerebral cortex is stimulated by electricity, one of the most frequent responses is eye movement. When parts of the left cerebral hemisphere are stimulated, the eyes move to the right. When parts of the right cerebral hemisphere are stimulated, the eyes move to the left. When asked a question, a person will characteristically look up and to one side as he ponders the answer. Although previously perceived as an idiosyncracy, as when teachers said, "Johnny, the answer is not on the ceiling"; we now know that left hemisphere functions will produce a right move of the eyes, and right hemisphere functions a left move of the eyes. People's eyes characteristically move in one direction or the other and they are, therefore, right movers or left movers, there being an equal number of each in the general population. (See Figure 2)

When a person moves his eyes to one side, he is activating one side of the brain for better concentration, and switching off the other. We all do this unconsciously when we must search our memory, solve mathematical problems mentally, or visualize. However, not all eye movements are perceptible, and

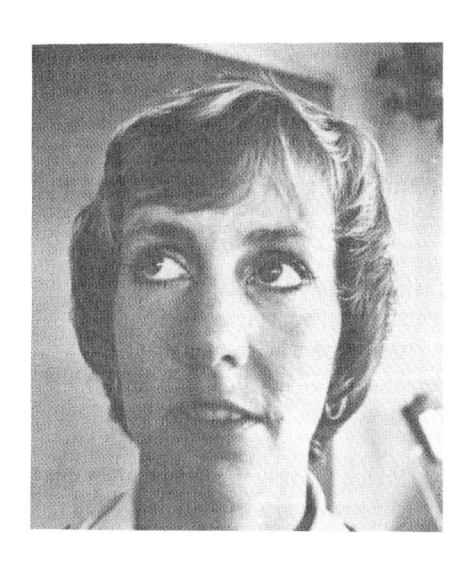

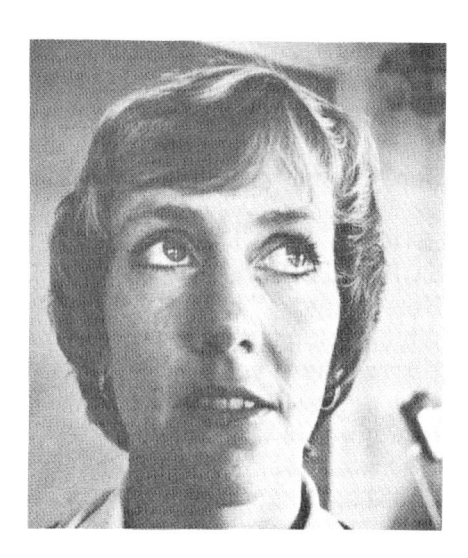

Fig. 2 When the left hemisphere is stimulated, the eyes move to the right. When the right hemisphere is stimulated, the eyes move to the left.

some people appear to always stare straight ahead. Muscle testing enables the examiner to detect which brain is switched-on and off. The side of the brain that is used most often, is the dominant brain. It usually corresponds to the brain which controls the dominant eye, but it may correspond to the brain which controls the dominant ear, or hand, or be totally different..

TECHNIQUE TO DETERMINE THE DOMINANT BRAIN
1. Test both right and left deltoid muscles in the clear.
2. Ask one of the questions or challenges listed below.
3. Observe the eye movements, if any. A right move will be a left brain response, a left move will be a right brain response.
4. Test each arm, one at a time, immediately following the response to your question. If both arms are still strong, both hemispheres were stimulated and an integrated response was given. If the left arm is weakened, and the right arm is strong, then the left brain was stimulated. If the right arm is weakened, and the left arm is strong, then the right brain was stimulated. The muscle test results should match the eye movements, if perceived by you.
5. If one side is repeatedly favored, no matter what the question, you may assume it to be dominant.

QUESTIONS OR CHALLENGES WHICH SWITCH ON ONE SIDE OF THE BRAIN ONLY.
1. How many "i's" in Mississippi?
2. Which color, red or green, is at the top of a traffic light?
3. Hum a tune to yourself.
4. How do you feel when you are angry?
5. How much is 12 times 13?
6. Who was President in 1942?
7. Count backwards from 100 to 1.
8. What is the difference between contraction and expansion?
9. Say 85193 backwards.
10. Draw a diamond shape.

VISUAL INTEGRATION
　　The relationship of eye movements to thinking starts early in life. The human organism begins to exist in space at birth and

learns how to use its eyes by moving toward or away from mother, food, sounds, and toys. At first, he may use each eye separately, but soon learns to use the eyes together as he learns to creep, crawl, walk and run. If he learns correct binocular eye movements, he will develop efficient visual skills for focusing near and far, depth perception, etc. If he does not learn these skills, he must compensate and "switch off" the message entering the brain to avoid the confusion of seeing double. The brain has a choice of integrating bilateral information or inhibiting it. If it does the latter, Energy is blocked and there is stress in the system.

VISUAL SWITCHING OFF

The visual field is approximately 180°. Each eye sees about 120° with an overlap or midline of about 60°. The left 90° is the left visual field and the right 90° is the right visual field. Although both cerebral hemispheres receive information from each eye, the left cerebral hemisphere is activated by looking toward the right visual field with the right eye leading. The right cerebral hemisphere is likewise activated by looking to the left.

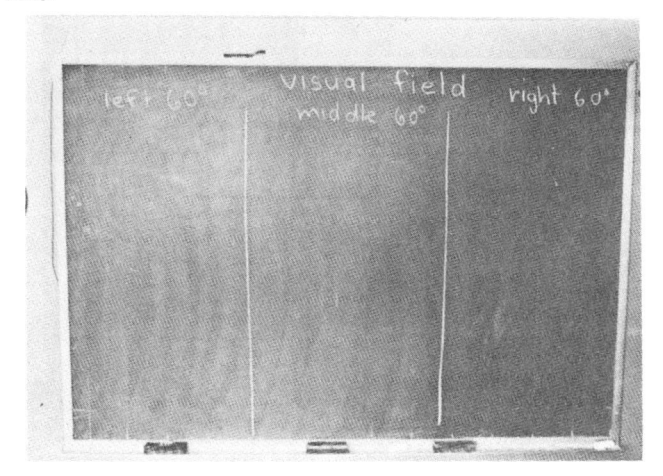

Fig. 3 The visual field is divided into right, left, and center by the Brain. Information from the left side goes directly to the right hemisphere. Information from the right goes directly to the left. The midline area, approximately 60°, is the area where hemispheric integration is necessary.

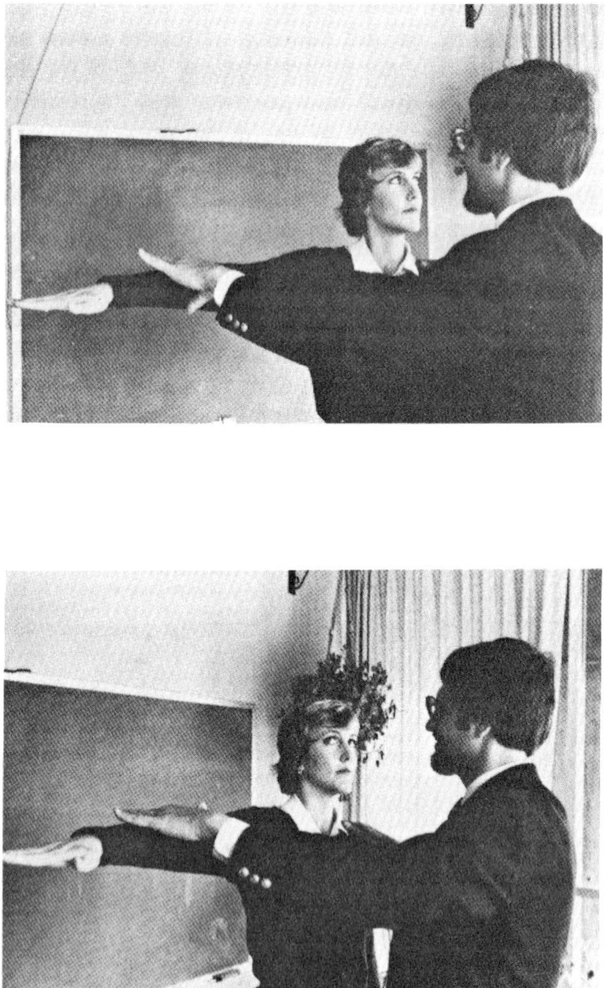

Fig. 4 Testing for visual integration, or switching off. Muscle testing when the eyes move to the right and left of the visual field reveals balance, or imbalance.

Edu-Kinesthetics uses muscle testing to determine the true quality of neurological organization, and to ascertain if there is sufficient integration for fluent learning. Like all muscle testing, these tests are simple as long as you understand the question you are asking the body. These tests involve muscle testing while instructing the subject to move the eyes and head in different directions.

TESTING FOR VISUAL INTEGRATION (See Figure 4)
1. Test a strong indicator muscle such as the Deltoid.
2. Ask the student to focus straight ahead at a target in the midline area. Hold the target at least eighteen inches away so that both eyes can focus on it. Unless there is a severe convergence problem, so that the person sees double, the muscle should test strong.
3. Now ask the student to look towards the left *without* moving the head. Does the muscle test strong, or weak?
4. Now ask the student to look towards the right; again watch for no head movement whatsoever. Does the muscle test strong, or weak?

IMPLICATIONS
1. If strong straight ahead, right, and left, there is good visual integration and no stress on the visual field.
2. If strong left and weak right, the student is probably left-eye dominant and right-brained. If there are learning problems, you are on the way to resolving them.
3. If strong to the right and weak to the left, there may not be severe problems, however, the student may read slowly and avoid near point tasks or have other complications. Again, he will be helped by you.

SWITCHING ON THE VISUAL SYSTEM
There are several techniques to switch on the system, depending upon the severity of the problem. You may use one or all of the following, the more the better. To find out if you have switched on your student, use the same muscle tests before and after the techniques chosen so that you and your student feel the difference. An immediate improvement in reading speed and comprehension may be experienced as well.

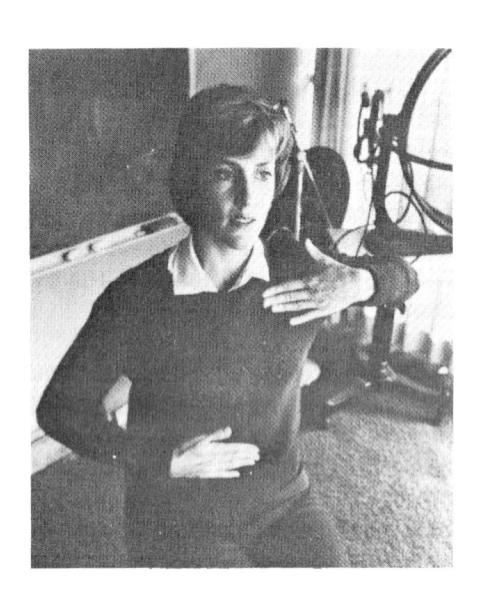

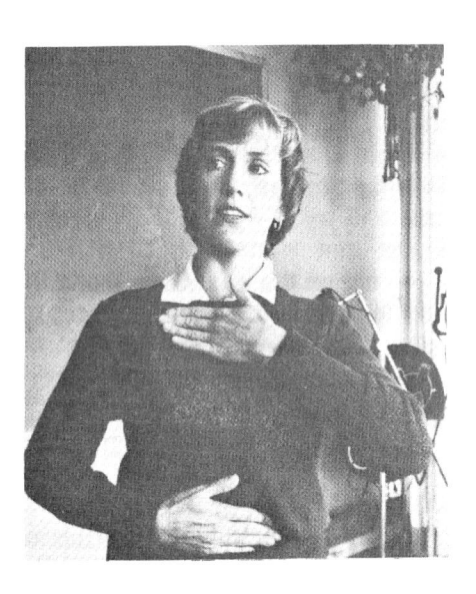

Fig. 5 Massaging the Kidney 27's, acupressure points located beneath the collar bone and to the right and left of the sternum, while resting the other hand on the navel.

1. *Cross-Crawl*
   Many cases need only cross-motor patterning to switch on the visual field. Cross-crawl exercises can balance the muscles, including the muscles controlling the eyes. So balance by cross-crawling prior to practicing the following eye exercises, and unnecessary switching off will soon stop. Use a penlight held 18 inches from the eyes for the following exercises:
   a) Pursuits or back-and-forth tracking through the entire visual field.
   b) Rotations—clockwise and counterclockwise circles around the entire visual field.
   c) Convergence exercises. Starting at 18 inches from the eyes, slowly push the penlight closer and closer toward the nose, watching the eyes. Stop when your student sees double or the eyes stop converging.
2. *Massage*
   Rub deeply and firmly the acupressure points known as Kidney 27's while holding one hand over the navel area. (See Figure 5)

   An ancient method of Energy balance is acupuncture and acupressure. Energy crosses over from one side of the body to the other when activated by these points. Homolateral crawlers will often spontaneously cross-crawl by switching on these points. Walther's book on Kinesiology states that these points are alternators which allow the flow of Energy from one side of the body to the other. He states further that "K 27 is classified by the Chinese in classic acupuncture as the 'home of the associated points.' It is the associated point of all the associated points."
3. *Yoga* (See Figure 6.)
   Relax the head and upper torso into a modified backbend, depending upon agility and flexibility. With head back, allow gravity to melt away the tension and breathe deeply to bring Energy into the neck. If chest is concave, attempt to open it without strain. Now move the eyes back and forth across the ceiling several times and keep breathing. There are proprioceptors in the neck muscles which switch on the eye muscles when the neck is in this position. This is the position of the neck during creeping and crawling when you first learned to use your eyes together as a team.

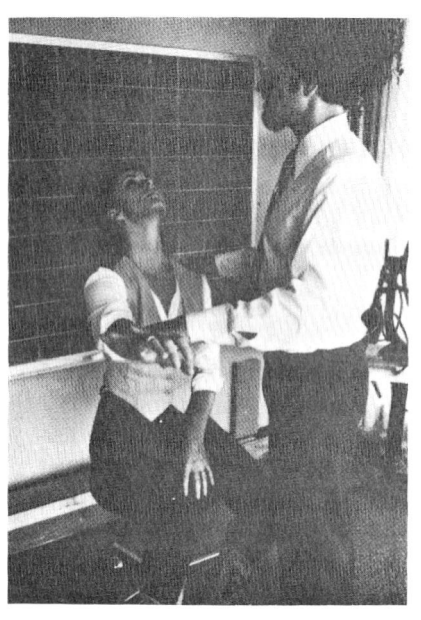

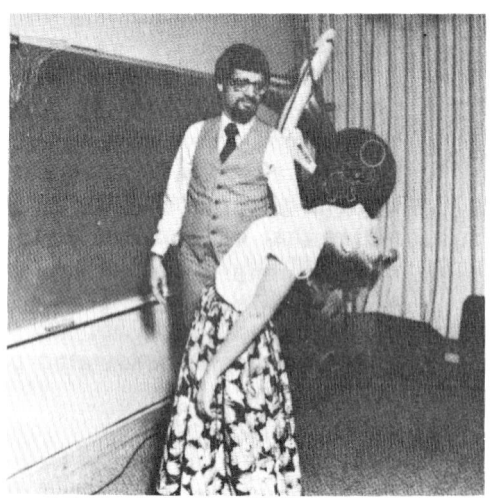

Fig. 6 Letting the head hang back without effort, while breathing deeply and rhythmically and rotating the eyes in either direction. The more backbend that can be accomplished, the better the results.

Edu-Kinesthetics maintains that "muscles have memories." As the neck was in this position when we first learned synchronized, switched-on eye movements, years later a return to this posture can switch them on again!

EDU-KINESTHETICS AND THE EARS

Listening and language development has been largely taken for granted, and, aside from hearing tests for those suspected of deafness, little intervention for listening instruction has ever been done. E-K and muscle testing introduces the concept of earedness, and provides a way to measure bilateral listening integration.

Recent brain research has demonstrated that, just as eyes move in the direction of a visual target, ears point in the direction of sound. A baby will turn its head toward noise, and proprioceptors again in the neck trigger the brain to switch on one ear or the other. (See Figure 7)

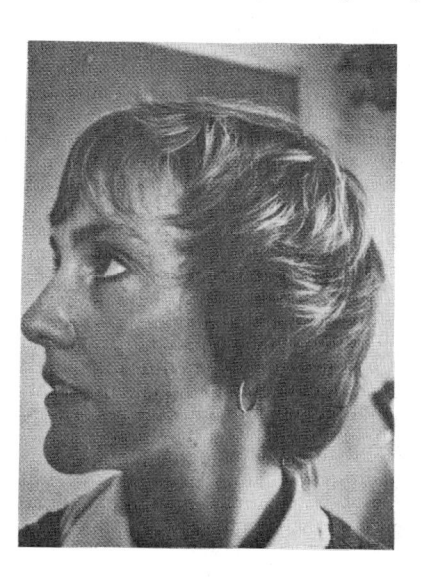

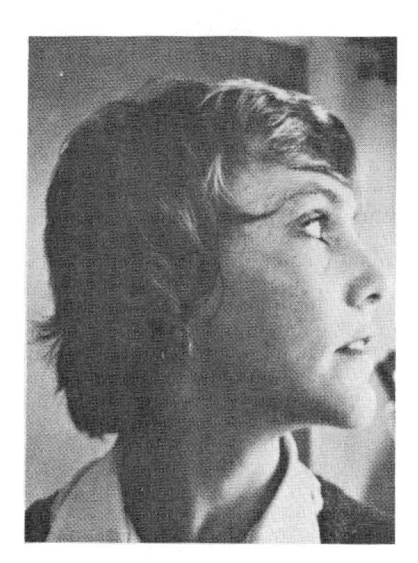

Fig. 7 When the left hemisphere is stimulated by sound, the head turns to the right. When the right hemisphere is stimulated by sound, the head turns to the left.

Again, like the eyes, the right brain has direct access to the left ear, and the left brain uses the right ear. Infants seem born with the capacity to listen to language, a left-brain function, with the right ear, and to listen to rhythms with the left ear, a right-brain function.

The dominant ear will generally correspond to the dominant eye and brain. Observing the direction of head turning can be informative. Some people have difficulty turning the head in one direction. This would be the nondominant side.

The muscle test for a switched-off ear is similar to the eyes, only now the student does turn the head.

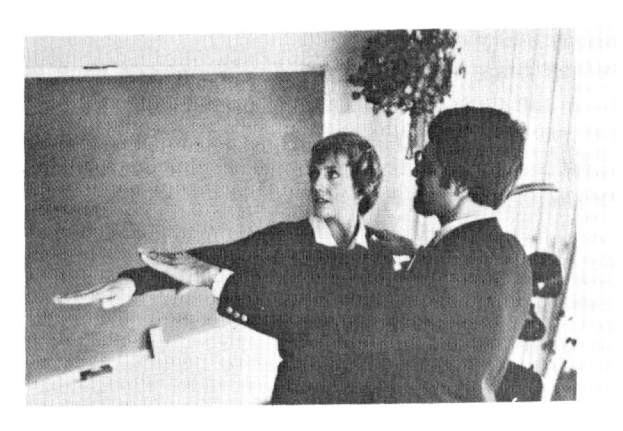

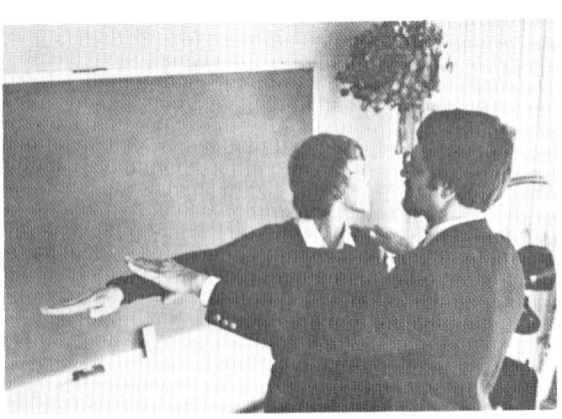

Fig. 8 Muscle testing, with the head turned to the right or left, reveals balance or imbalance in the energy flow for listening abilities.

MUSCLE TEST FOR EAR BALANCE AND AUDITORY INTEGRATION (See Figure 8)
1. Select a strong indicator muscle and test the student facing straight ahead.
2. Now ask the student to turn his head to the right. Is the indicator muscle strong, or weak?
3. Now test the student turning to the left.

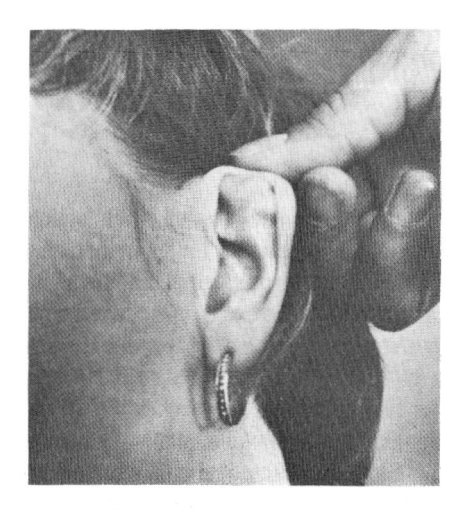

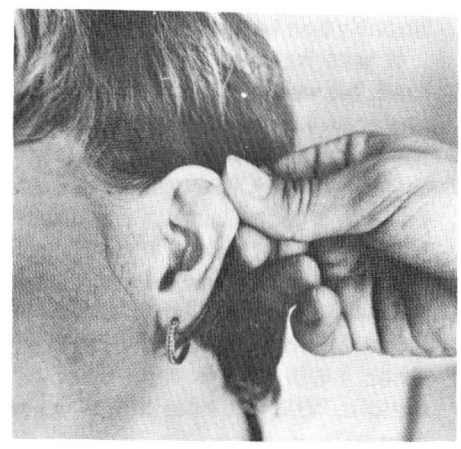

Fig. 9 Folding the ears back, starting from the top and working down, brings energy to the ears, and listening skills improve.

IMPLICATIONS
1. If strong turning to both right and left sides, there is good auditory integration.
2. If weak when turning right, but strong when turning left, the student is probably right-brained for auditory functions with below average auditory attention, memory, and listening abilities. You will be able to help him.
3. If weak turning left, but strong when turning right, the student is extremely left-brained for auditory functions and he may read slowly, without rhythm and phrasing, and he may also have poor speech development and speak in a monotone. You will be able to help him, also.

SWITCHING ON THE EARS (See Figure 9)

Fold the ears back, starting from the top down. This brings Energy to the ears, and listening and language skills improve.

This auricular exercise is known to bring energy to the body by people involved in muscle balancing work. I discovered its relationship to language when working with Jeffrey, a boy who has been virtually deaf since birth. He learned to speak using a technique whereby he placed his hand on his mother's throat and imitated the vibrational frequency when activating his own throat muscles. Often such deaf speakers have a distinctive rhythm, pitch, and phrasing. However, Jeffrey can speak quite fluently and has total expressive language abilities.

It was noticed by parents and teachers that when Jeffrey read, his voice would change. It would get a high, nasal sound and lose all rhythmic and expressive qualities. Giving Jeffrey the usual E-K examination customary at the time, I was unable to balance him through cross-crawling, K 27's, or the breathing and yoga techniques. Remembering the auricular exercise of folding back the ears, I tried this on Jeffrey as a last resort. The response was immediate. His eyes focused, his muscles strengthened and, what was most exciting, his reading voice changed! He could now read with his natural, right-brained, voice. I will always remember Jeffrey's mother shouting with delight, "Did you hear that? Do you hear him reading? I love it! I love it!"

I have since discovered the importance of earedness and of switching on the ears of all people who switch off.

PLEASE TAKE SPECIAL NOTICE

The human brain defies simplistic analysis, so this information is used, together with other educational test data and common sense for the intention of helping people. Language develops in both sides of the brain prior to age five and there is much overlap of stored information in both brains in some people whose brains do not specialize. Also, many left-handed and crossed dominant people store language skill in the right brain and the many right brain skills in the left. If you are aware of this, these tests will help you to spot these people.

DENNISON LATERALITY CHECKLIST

Name _____ Date _____

Dominance	*Check Correct Choice*	*Determined by* (check one or more)
Hand	Right Left Ambidexterous	1. Observation 2. Interview
Eye	Right Left Mixed	1. Looking through hole 2. Muscle testing 3. Eye movements 4. Observation
Ear	Right Left Mixed	1. Head movements 2. Muscle testing
Brain	Right Left	1. Observation 2. Muscle testing 3. Eye movements 4. Head movements

This checklist includes the methods found most helpful by Edu-Kinesthetics. The information is used to determine the areas which need balancing. Consistency of movement, and integrated strategies when thinking and problem solving, is the ultimate goal.

PROLOGUE TO
CHAPTER VIII

TWO EXTREME OPPOSITES—BRAIN LEFT AND BRAIN RIGHT

The heroes of this fantasy are two strange, but distinct individuals. They are as different as night and day, yet they attend the same schools, travel to the same places, and apply for the same jobs, as if they were alike. They are unaware of each other's existence, although they *need each other* more than each will ever know. They both play a significant and equal role in resolving the conflict presented in the plot of this book. To fully appreciate how an age-old mystery can be solved, the reader is forewarned to know these people extremely well. To preserve the anonymity of our subjects, we will call them Brain Left and Brain Right for reasons which will become clear as we proceed.

Brain Left goes through life like a computer, and even looks like one. He never gets very excited about anything, but he is capable of processing and storing vast amounts of data efficiently and methodically, one step at a time. Brain Left prefers auditory information, especially spoken language, and stores it in a logical and organized fashion for subsequent retrieval. When asked to speak, he will regurgitate data in the monotonous, electronic voice of a robot. He prints and writes data stiffly and mechanically, following encoded rules of line, sequence and grammatical structure, but he cannot draw, and is never creative nor artistic. Brain Left can concentrate on a single item or problem beautifully and will "tune out" all distractions until he is sure he has figured out the correct answer. He prefers to analyze and reason logically rather than trust intuition and follow a "hunch." His satisfactions come from efficiency, order, and mathematical exactitude. He is tense, rigid, and clumsy moving in space, and can make a fool of himself on the dance floor. He has no interest in participating in sports and, frankly, avoids moving and touching whenever possible. He would rather sit and think.

Brain Right perceives the universe as a whole, and senses the fullness and completeness of all the dimensions of experience. She would never dream of trying to understand or make a logical analysis of a problem. Brain Right would simply "know" the truth and trust its rightness. Brain Right might be called an artist. She is intensely curious about her material environment and lives the present moment to the fullest! She uses her eyes and ears to store pictures to paint and melodies to sing. She is forever the three-year-old in her rediscovery of the beauty of the world around her. Her imagination is unbounded and she can recall and construct visual information easily. She rejects auditory information processing, and gets confused by tasks involving too many steps which she must remember. She is governed by her emotions, and can go from ecstasy to despair in a moment. Always the actor and a real "ham," if you feed her a line, she will steal the show. Her voice is so expressive of the meaning of the words, and her hands and body communicate meaning as well. She feels the meaning of life, and she makes others "feel" too.

Brain Right is a good athlete and is well-coordinated in all her movements through space. Her actions seem relaxed and effortless, for she is in perfect tune with her body. She is a terrific dancer, too, for she can really get into the music.

Brain Right is a horrible reader and an atrocious speller. She can copy letters as if they were designs, but cannot write or recognize them by name. She can recognize faces, but not words, unless they happen to be highly meaningful, such as a commercial trademark. She has little use for the sound-symbol relationship necessary for most modern Western languages. She remembers and recognizes numbers more easily.

Brain Right is aware of her total environment, and performs by instinct, often appearing to be undisciplined, impetuous and unable to concentrate. She is uncomfortable in schools that restrict her freedom to move and may blurt out answers.

She is bored by seat work, mental tricks, puns, and puzzles.

No one exists who fits these two extremes exactly as described. However you are probably all too well acquainted with people similar to Brain Right or Brain Left already. Do you know people like them? Do these profiles make you suspicious or downright nervous that one of them may be lurking within you?

Someone like Brain Left would be a good listener. He makes order out of chaos and can live in apparent confusion, for his order is internal. He does not mind living in the city, working in a large office, hearing loud music, nor seeing an untidy house. As long as he can talk to himself, he is happy.

Someone like Brain Right, however, must have order to function. Too much conflicting sound or visual disharmony gets her confused and spoils her concentration. She cannot cope with noise and clutter. She needs an attractive, quiet and peaceful environment in order to relax and visualize.

Someone like Brain Left can remember what he hears and can speak without notes.

Someone like Brain Right requires careful planning and review if she is to talk. She may take copious notes and keep records and files. In contrast to a person like Brain Left, who takes essay exams without hesitation, trusting memory to relinquish the necessary information, the Brain Right type would prefer to recognize the answers on a multiple-choice test.

Although we can recognize people who remind us of Brain Right and Brain Left, no one functions entirely like either in real life (except after certain surgical procedures or strokes). People can function like Brain Right and Brain Left, however, when under stress and that is why recognizing these behaviors is important.

CHAPTER VIII
A SWITCHED-ON BRAIN!

In order to understand the role of the brain in learning the skills of reading, writing, spelling, and math, it is useful to think of a switch on a household appliance—a vacuum cleaner, for example. When we turn the switch to "on," it works. But what really happens? First, a desicion is made to switch it on. When we do, Energy, in the form of electricity, flows from a power source, the power plant, to a motor which is designed, or programmed to perform a certain function (turn wheels, drive belts, etc.). When the function is no longer needed, we switch it off, terminating our message to the machine.

The relationship of our brain and body is exactly the same. When the brain decides what work needs to be done, our body is a fantastic machine which receives messages through the nervous system. When we want to pick up a glass, that decision in the brain sends power to the muscle to do so. The muscle contracts when we switch on the signal and relaxes when we switch it off. The brain is constantly switching messages on and off to all the muscles and organs of the body. Most of these decisions are automatic and involuntary. We could not possibly function if we had to consciously think about the regulation of our heartbeat, breathing, digestion, etc. We take this switching on and off for granted, unless something goes wrong.

THE HUMAN BRAIN

Our brain should really be called our "brains," as we all have two unique and specialized minds controlling our bodies and sorting knowledge for future decision-making. These two brains are known as Hemispheres; the Left Hemisphere is mainly in charge of the right side of the body, and the Right Hemisphere is mainly in charge of the left. They are interconnected by the Corpus Callosum, a bundle of nerve fibers. A complex system of switches is developed in infancy to synchronize and integrate information so that the two brains can work together in harmony and coordination. Hemispheres can take over for each other when necessary, and one may operate its own side for a given task. In general, the more complex the task, the more both sides of the brain may be involved in the operation. (See Figure 1)

The two halves of the brain, in addition to their separate responsibilities of switching on and off the physical body, have separate functions regarding consciousness and thought processes. A Duality seems intrinsic in the Universe, be it Day versus Night, Yin versus Yang, Mind versus Intuition, Logic versus Art, or Left versus Right. It appears that the brain too, is so divided. The Left Hemisphere is predominantly involved in the analytical thinking, especially language and logic. It gets switched-on when we need to process computer-like information with sequence and structure. The Right Hemisphere, in contrast, is responsible for our visual memory, orientation in space, artistic ability, feeling and emotions, body awareness and recognition of faces. It gets switched-on when we need to process information as a whole, simultaneously, rather than in linear fashion.

It is becoming increasingly more popular to talk about Right and Left Brain. We read research studies and hear enlightened discussions. Everyone seems familiar with the concept that there is a difference between the two Hemispheres of the brain. Most of us, even those of us in the field, have not thought very much beyond this point.

After fifteen years of research and experimentation with students, E-K now provides a method for understanding what is going on in the brain which the layperson and professional can use for practical purposes. We are excited about this, because it works and makes sense, and because it explains much of what had been elusive over the years. We do not sug-

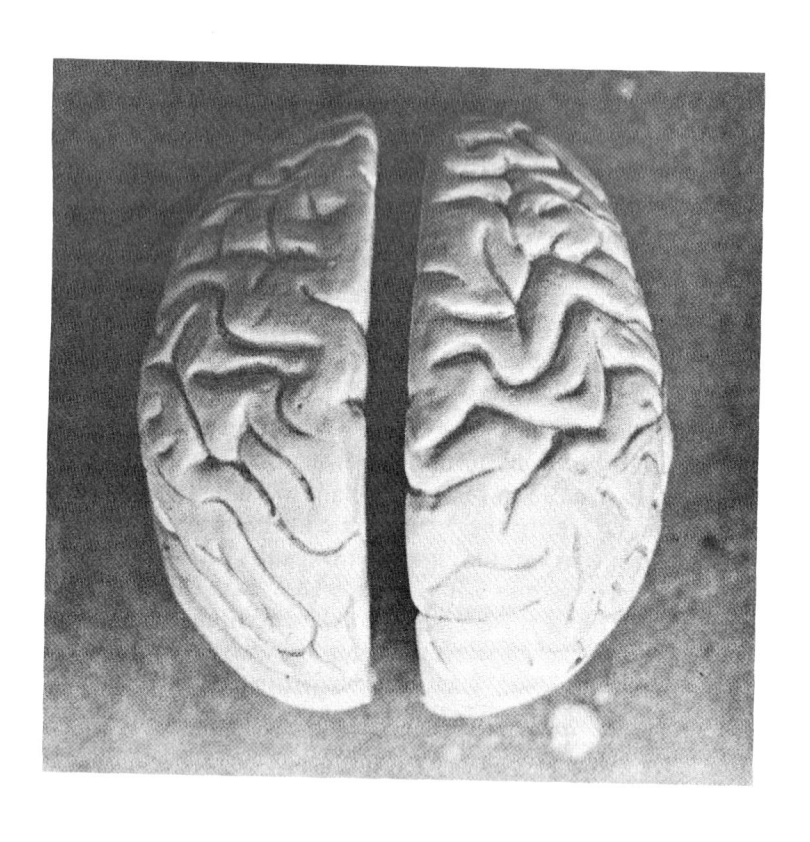

Fig. 1 The right hemisphere and the left hemisphere of the brain are two totally separate and distinct organs, connected only by a bundle of nerve fibers called the Corpus Callosum.

gest that we have all the answers however, our concept of the brain is so useful, manageable, and predictable, that we feel we are "three giant steps" ahead and the results we are getting, with both normal and retarded children, is incredible.

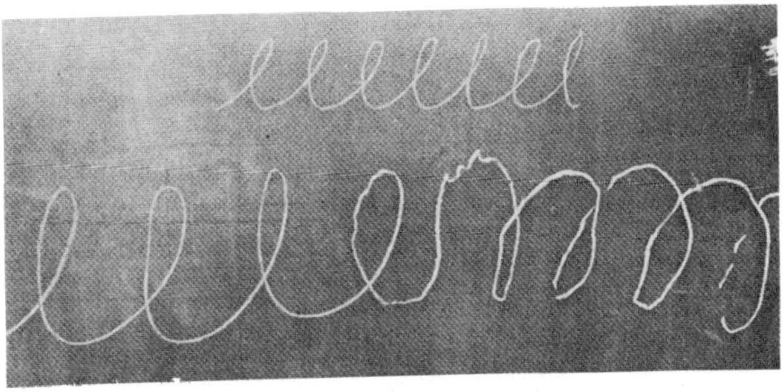

Fig. 2 Jimmy copied the top series of loops while standing at the center of the chalkboard.

Considerable stress and indecision were observed at the midpoint, however, Jimmy was unaware that he had changed the direction of his loops. What made this happen? Why couldn't Jimmy see that right and left were not alike? Couldn't he feel that the loops were different when he drew them? What happened when he got to the middle? Is this Dyslexia?

Figure 3 is a simplified sketch of the two sides or Hemispheres of the brain when a person has hemispheric integration. The arrows represent nerve pathways to show how visual images are processed from the eye to the brain.

Figure 4 is a picture of what apparently happened as Jimmy processed the task of drawing his loops. Study the picture and pretend to be Jimmy for a few moments and it will help you understand the complex processes which we take for granted.

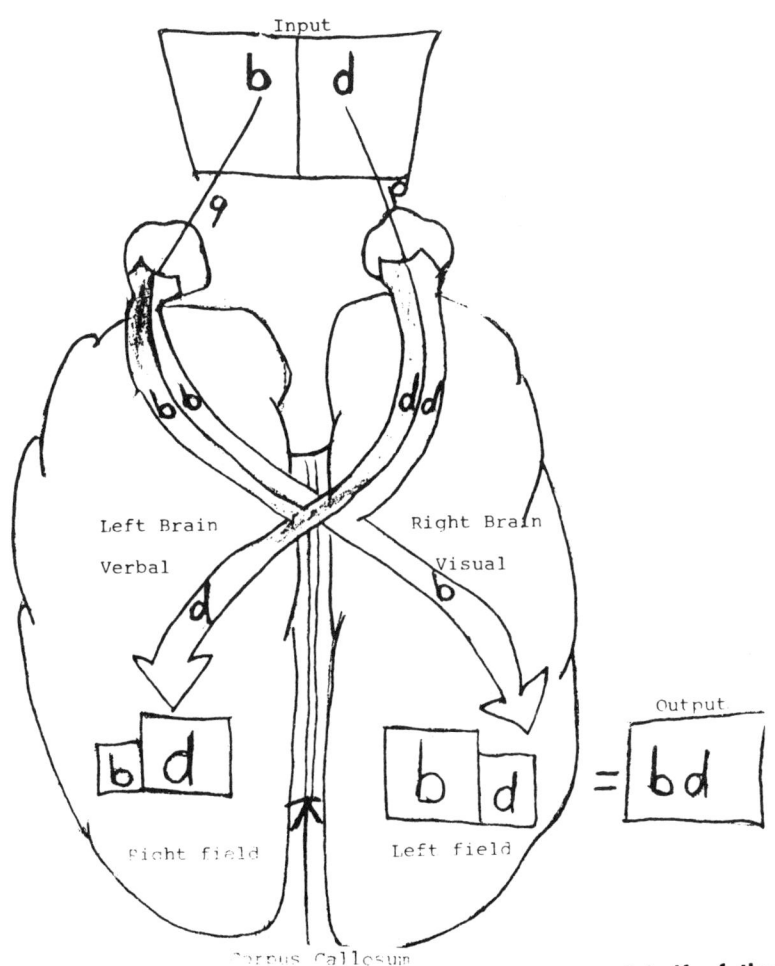

Fig. 3 Nerve pathways in a normal person connect half of the visual field to each hemisphere. Feedback via the Corpus Callosum from the other hemisphere is necessary for efficient processing of information (represented by the smaller squares). The Left Brain receives information directly from the right eye (darker arrow), and indirectly from the right via the Corpus Callosum, which connects the two sides for this purpose. Likewise, the Right Brain receives information directly from the left eye, and indirectly from the right. The Right Brain processes visually as a whole. The Left Brain analyzes and processes bits of information through language and logic.

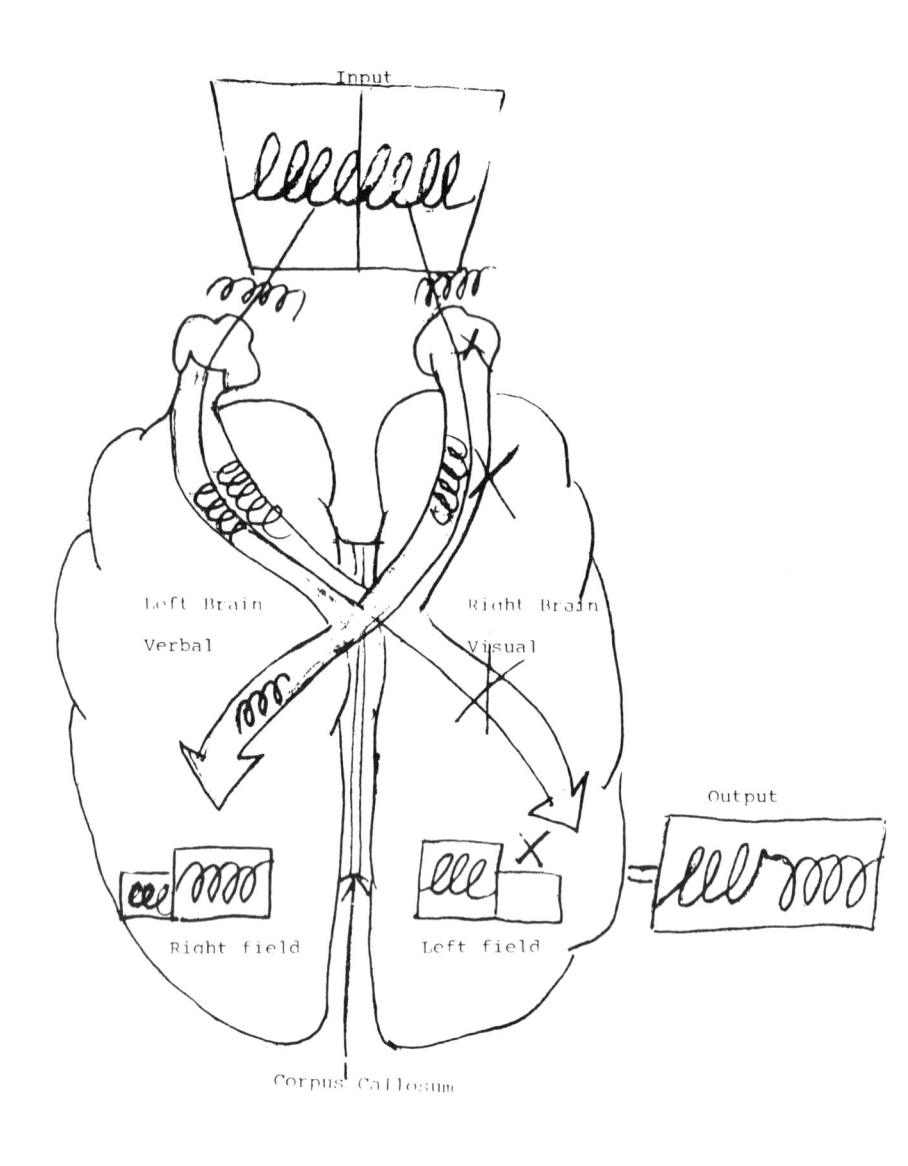

Fig. 4 Switched off nerve pathways to right brain result in confusion as feedback from right brain is not available after crossing midline into the right field. Incorrect left brain information predominates.

This is how Edu-Kinesthetics enables us to understand and work with Jimmy:
1. Jimmy is left-eye dominant and Right-Brain dominant. This is determined by muscle testing. When he points his eyes to the left, he is strong. When he points his eyes to the right, he is weak. When he listens with his left ear (connected to the Right Brain also) he is strong. When listening with the right ear, he is weak.
2. When he commences to draw the pattern, his Right Brain is on and strong, as he functions well with the left eye in the left visual field. His Right Brain is in charge and he is happy and aware of his body.
3. When he reaches the midpoint or midline of his body, where synchronization and binocular focusing of the two eyes is essential, there is conflict as the two brains have not learned to work together in the right field. The Left Brain should take over, translating the outside-in movement going toward the midline into an inside-out movement going away from the midline intellectually, while the Right Brain provides visual feedback, keeping Jimmy aware of the whole while he concentrates on the part.
4. Instead, Jimmy tries too hard. He switches off (confirmed by muscle testing) the Right Brain, his strong dominant mode, in order to zero in and concentrate upon using the Left Brain. His Right Brain actually goes into an alpha brain wave, meditational state, as he deals with the stress of crossing the midline and using the right eye and working in the right visual field. An EEG or VER would show a pattern similar to a person with a blind left eye.
5. Instead of seeing and drawing the pattern the way the Right Brain would see it from the left eye, he gets back the reciprocal image indirectly via the Corpus Callosum and lacks the feedback-feed-forward mechanism to correct himself. The image on the retina is actually upside down. Unaccustomed to using this left brain, right eye alone, he is confused by this. It is our experience moving in space, a Right Brain skill, which teaches us to perceive what we see.

The explanation of Jimmy's experience acquaints us with the concepts crucial to understanding and working with the two Hemispheres of the brain:

1. There are two separate brains, Right and Left, involved in our perception of physical reality.
2. The two brains are either working together, or they are in conflict. Conflict may lead to inefficient information processing and switching off.
3. The two brains perceive information in totally and completely different manners. We must understand the consciousness of each to learn effectively.
4. Awareness of the total visual field, and ability to work on each side of, and across the midline, is fundamental.
5. Concentration must be stress free, so that we do not switch off one side of the brain. We must always be aware that the "whole is more than the sum of its parts."
6. The right brain is vital to our physical performance.

In order to help ourselves or others to learn, grow, or change, we have to know how we operate. Just as some plants need more sun and others need more water, people have individual needs, which must be identified.

TWO LEARNING TYPES

Edu-Kinesthetics provides a unique method for easily diagnosing and identifying two different major learning types. All people fall within these groups, and, when identified, the characteristics of people within the groups are similar. Once it is determined whether we switch-off the right or left brain, a positive plan of action can be set into motion that will work, instead of trial-and-error or well-intentioned efforts to fit a square peg into a round hole.

It is fun, and it would be useful, to discover your own pattern of neurological organization. Work together with your partner to find out which type you are and what type he is. Does it seem to fit your personalities? Does this explain anything to you that you always wondered about?

The concept of the two cerebral hemispheres has been well developed. (See chapter VII) Are you auditory, or visual? The auditory learner uses left-brained thinking, sounds out words, spells phonetically, is verbal, logical, and prefers to follow rules. The visual learner uses right-brained thinking, and prefers sight reading and spelling, and is creative and intuitive in problem-solving. Without muscle testing, however, it has not been as simple as it may sound to classify a person due to the complexities of neurological organization.

The two types of learners are identified by: 1) establishing a dominant Cerebral Hemisphere, right or left, and 2) establishing which hemisphere is switched-off, if any, when under the stress of reading, writing, spelling, or speaking, and by observing what happens around the midline.

Now suppose you were dyslexic and did not read and write as a child. You had some artistic talent, and became a painter because you were accepted at an art school. You spent fifteen years of your life trying to paint before you realized that you are a writer and prefer a verbal medium to a visual one. A simple muscle test confirms that painting requires a switching off of the dominant left brain, creating stress, while writing establishes balance, enabling both hemispheres to cooperate in harmony. This is what happened to a close family member. Edu-Kinesthetics has helped him make some decisions in his life that he felt were right and are now confirmed.

Another case is the hard-working student who overcame his Dyslexia through perseverance and determination. Convinced that he could succeed in school, he "showed them" by studying for years and earning a Ph.D. Assumed auditory, because he did not do neat art work as taught by art teachers, and because he was a good writer, he pursued a highly verbal learning career. A simple muscle test would have shown that he was a right-brained, visual learner. He could do the left-brained, auditory work, but at the expense of repressed creativity and fluency. In his case, myopia, poor posture, and tension resulted. This is my profile, and I am, fortunately, better integrated today by learning to let go, relax, and switch on my right brain.

Do you switch off the right brain, or the left brain? Edu-Kinesthetics suggests that most people growing up in the Twentieth Century, modern, industrial world, fall into a pattern similar to my own. We learn to try too hard and switch off the right brain when under pressure.

The chapter on writing will shed more light on the subject of right and left brain and is a continuation of this discussion.

The two lists below help us compare the functions and thinking of each brain. As you study these words, think about how each is the exact and total opposite of the other across the page.

CHARACTERISTICS OF LEFT AND RIGHT BRAINS

Left Brain	*Right Brain*
Auditory	Visual
Myopic	Hyperopic
Convergent	Divergent
Analytic	Synthetic
Abstract	Concrete
Rational	Emotional
Temporal	Spatial
Digital	Analogic
Objective	Subjective
Active	Passive
Tense	Relaxed
Euphoric	Depressed
Sympathetic	Parasympathetic
Propositional	Appositional
Sequential-Linear	Gestalt-Simultaneous
Mental	Intuitive
Scientific	Artistic
Logical	Psychic
Introvert	Extrovert

Why I Hate to Write

I hate to write because it usuall comes in the form of paragras or storys.

Most paragraphs come in the form of punishment. Punishment writing come in 1000 word bulks on subjects like ball bounys or shoe laces.

The last reason is reading it or having some one else read it is that the might not be able to read it or understand it. The best part of ~~writ~~ writing a paragraph is finishing it.

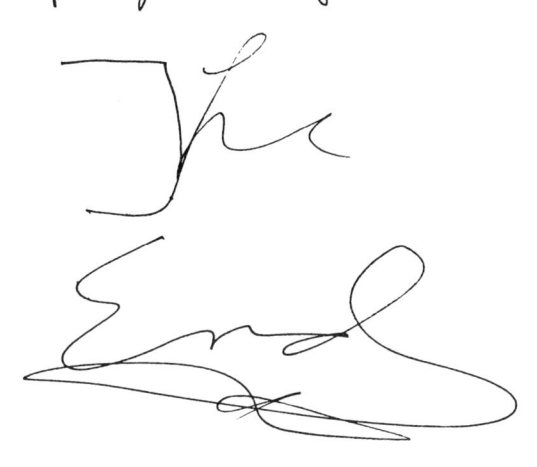

The End

CHAPTER IX

WRITING ANALYSIS

After Ruth and I exchanged our usual greetings and I felt she was sufficiently relaxed and at ease to start our session, I said, "Take out your pencil and paper, and we will have a little spelling test." The changes in her body were immediate and obvious. The stress signs were all there. Her skin paled, her brow wrinkled, her jaw tightened and her right shoulder dropped as she got into a posture for writing. Her head turned to the right and she leaned back to the left. Holding the pencil in her right hand, she turned the paper so that she would be writing in a vertical line perpendicular to her body. As she wrote, she was able to keep the left side of her body immobile. The only movement, other than in her right hand and arm, were various facial contortions as she watched what she was doing out of the right eye. (See Figure 1)

Handwriting analysis has for years been offered as a way to unlock the secrets of the writer's mind, health, and personality. Much can be learned from a sample of handwriting, but that is not the intent of this chapter. Handwriting analysis makes use of the product of one's handwriting. Edu-Kinesthetics is interested in the process. We use muscle testing and trained observations to gain insights into what is happening within the writer in order to get symbols down on paper!

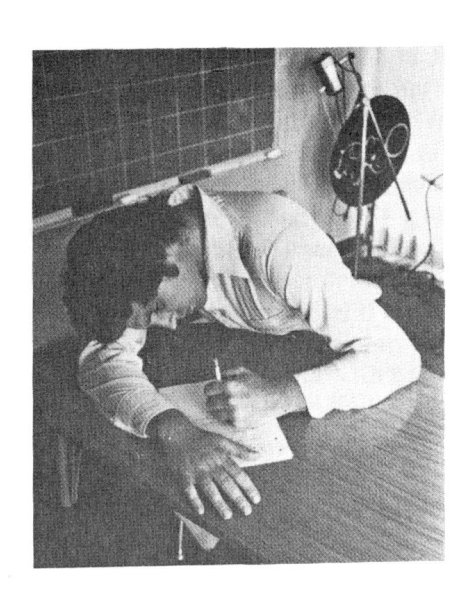

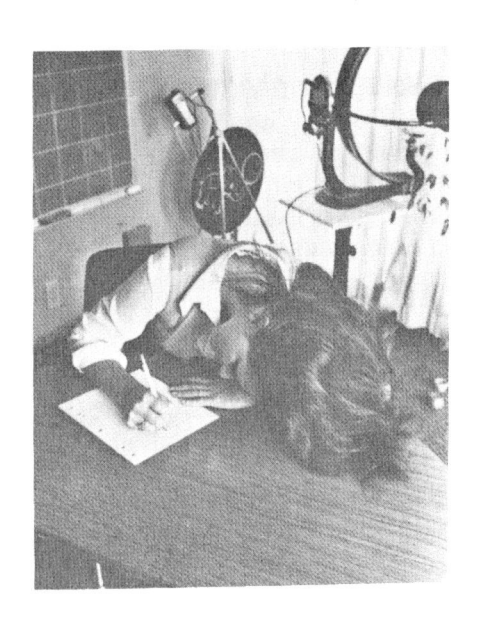

Fig. 1 The posture of the writer must be recognized as a symptom of stress on the information processing system.

Edu-Kinesthetics believes that, in most cases, a skilled analysis of posture, movement, and visual habits while writing, and a positively reinforced reprogramming of switched-off writing habits into switched-on habits hold the key to learning. The main theme of this book is that reading and writing must be expressive acts to be successful. A reading problem is a writing problem, and correcting these has more to do with "switching on" the expressive language of the child than memorizing words or studying phonics workbooks. Edu-Kinesthetics will show you how simple it is to understand and correct a learning problem before it gets serious, and how to turn around a person with an advanced disability. All that is needed is a commitment to change, an E-K balanced environment, and some loving patience.

In this chapter you will learn to:
1. Observe a "switched-off" posture.
2. Analyze visual field performance.
3. Use muscle testing to help another person internalize a "switched-on" posture.
4. Use muscle testing to determine if learning is taking place in both the Right and Left Brain.

HANDEDNESS AND WRITING ABILITY

The skill of writing, like reading, is a manmade invention which requires a certain degree of adaptation to learn. Some find learning to write easy; others do not. Misconceptions about the role of handedness and dominance in writing have caused untold misery and hardship to millions of children and have compromised the potential of millions of others. We all know that it is a right-handed world, and we know that most people write with their dominant right hand. The dominant hand performs better because the dominant brain, in this case the left brain, exerts conscious control over it. This is fine, when such control is needed, as when first learning to write. However, E-K maintains that, once learned, writing must become a right-brain controlled task, irregardless of handedness and dominance. Writing requires free movement, fluency, and expressiveness, and must be in tune with the flow of Energy in the body. Writing must be automatic, rhythmic, and beyond the need of much conscious control, like breathing. For balanced writing, the right brain, and not the left brain, must control the right hand. When the left brain is paying too much attention to the writing, when it should be attending to the thoughts to be communicated, switched-off writing and spelling result. Understanding the developmental process of writing skills helps to explain how this switching-off is learned by so many people.

COUNTERCLOCKWISE ENERGY

Neurologists, psychologists, and some educators have known for decades that when children are ready to read, between the mental ages of 5½ and 7½, they begin to form circles in a counterclockwise direction when they write. It is the children who do not do this who have the problem. Edu-Kinesthetics recognizes that this counterclockwise motion is right brain Energy moving toward the left, much in the same way that the right brain turns the head and the eyes to the left. When the child feels this need to draw in counterclockwise motions, his right brain is showing that it is ready to take over writing from the left brain so that the latter can think about the language, sounds and the verbal message. Hemispheric specialization is taking place as the child matures. Prior to this time, both hemispheres did everything. From this point forward, specialization is necessary for the complexity of information processing.

To prove the power of the counterclockwise circle on Energy balance, perform the following muscle test on your student-partner:
1. Muscle test a strong indicator muscle.
2. Ask student to draw a circle. (Either in the air, on paper, or chalkboard)
3. Observe if it was drawn clockwise, or counterclockwise.
4. Muscle test the indicator muscle.
5. If clockwise, did the muscle weaken?
6. If counterclockwise, did the muscle stay strong?
7. Instruct student to draw a circle again, this time in the opposite direction.
8. Muscle test and note the results this time.

THE LAZY 8

All writing, whether seeing it, or feeling it, is perceived within the visual field much like an 8 on its side, or a "lazy 8." This configuration fills the entire field, with the crossing point coming at the center, or midline, which is the area where Right

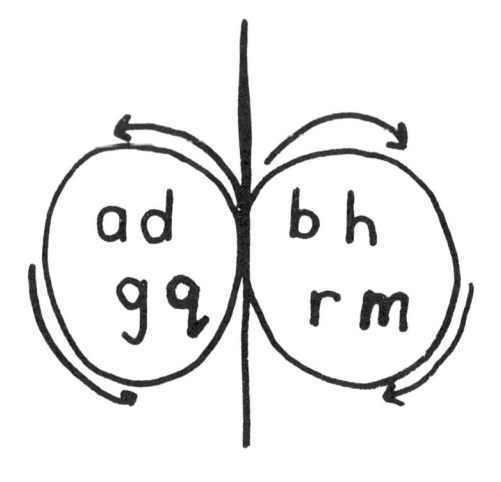

Fig. 2 The "lazy 8" conforms to our visual field, with the centerline the starting point for all drawing and letters. When energy moves counterclockwise, first, from the center, the writer stays balanced. When energy moves clockwise, the writer is out of balance. Letters such as a, d, and g must start with a counterclockwise movement. Letters like b, h, and r start with the down stroke, then can move clockwise.

and Left Brain must be integrated and come together. If we call the center the starting point, the printing of letters either starts here moving counterclockwise (a, d, g, q) or starts here with a downstroke, then moving clockwise (l, r, h, m). By superimposing them in your mind, all letters can be integrated into the "lazy 8." (See Figure 2)

To prove the power of the "lazy 8" with muscle testing, perform the following experiments with your student-partner:

"LAZY 8" MUSCLE TEST
1. Muscle test a strong indicator muscle in the clear.
2. Ask your student to trace a "lazy 8" in the air, moving clockwise from the center.
3. Muscle test the person. Does he test strong or weak?
4. If weak, draw the "lazy 8" again, this time in a counterclockwise movement from the center.
5. Muscle test the person again. Does he test strong again?

"LAZY 8" MUSCLE TEST FOR LETTERS
1. Muscle test a strong indicator muscle.
2. Instruct student to print any lower case letter.
3. Does he test weak after printing it?
4. Find a letter, if any, which, if he prints it, produces weakness.
5. If you get a weak response, does he print it in conformity to the "lazy 8" Energy flow?
6. If he does not print a letter correctly, instruct him to superimpose it upon the "lazy 8," and muscle test him again. Do you feel the difference in strength?

We have been doing this test with adults, and the responses in my seminars have been overwhelmingly positive and enlightening. People say things like, "Now I won't spell my name wrong anymore," and, "I always had to stop and think when I got to that letter."

POSTURE AND WRITING
To determine if someone switches off when writing, observe first the writer's posture. If the person is like Ruth or one of the other illustrations, he probably writes to the left or right of the midline. His body is saying, "I learned to write with my Left Brain and I still use the same posture I used when I was in

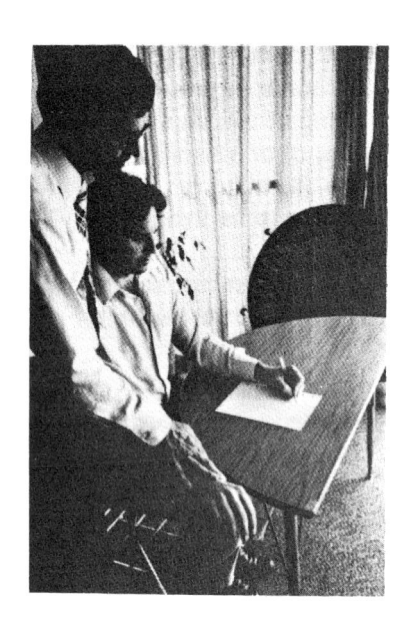

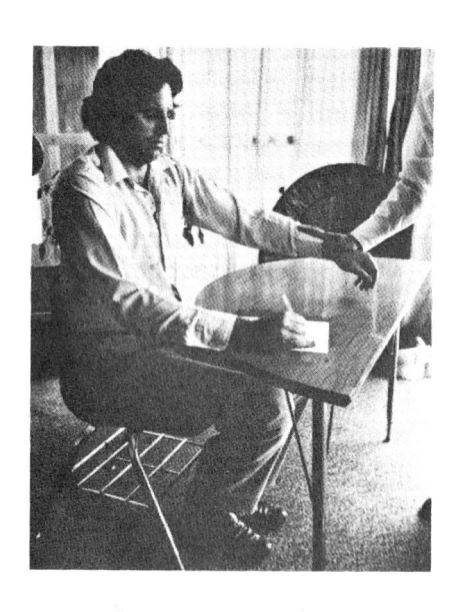

Fig. 3 A muscle test during the writing lesson will "lock-in" correct posture through positive reinforcement, or reveal imbalances.

grade school when my O's were never round enough." This posture requires the eyes to focus on the paper from different distances, and may have already resulted in vision problems for the individual.

If you suspect a "switched-off" writing posture, use muscle testing to confirm your suspicions:

TEST FOR A SWITCHED-OFF WRITING POSTURE
1. Test an indicator muscle to determine if it is strong.
2. Instruct your student to write a brief sentence.
3. Muscle test your student.
4. Does he test weak?
5. If weak, something caused him to switch off.

To correct a switched-off writing posture, modify the aspects of his posture to conform closer to the ideal as you feel it should be for him. Consult the illustrations in Figure 3. Move the paper more toward the middle if he has placed it to the side. Instruct him to keep his head up, about eighteen inches from the page. Change the angle of the paper if he has turned it sideways in order to write in a vertical line. Modify his grip on the pencil. It should be held loosely and the hand should be inverted so that both eyes can see the pencil point. When he writes in the corrected position and finds the ideal posture, he will muscle test strongly. The discovery of this writing imbalance and its correction through muscle testing is so dramatic to the student that, in many cases, the change to switched-on writing is permanent after only one demonstration!

Once a person has been "switched on" to learning and has internalized that success through a strong muscle test, the skilled facilitator will continue to "lock in" all balanced learning with strong muscle tests. There is no better positive reinforcement. (See Figure 3)

CHAPTER X

SWITCH ON TO READING

Ralph, age ten, cannot seem to remember a word from one line to the next. He tries so hard to read, but he just cannot learn. He can say the words on flash cards, or a list, but forgets everything when he has to read his book. Phonics, trying to sound out a word, is really difficult, too. He knows the sounds, but cannot remember them long enough to recognize a word containing the sound.

Brenda, age thirteen, appears to read beautifully. She performs with rhythm and inflection in her voce, and emphasizes all the right places. To hear her read orally, one would expect her to be the top reader in her class, but Brenda's comprehension is extremely poor. She cannot explain the main idea of a paragraph in her own words. She recalls only a few literal details, and often misunderstands. She cannot write a simple sentence, her spelling is atrocious, and she is dumbfounded if she must learn a new word out of context.

Ralph and Brenda are representative of millions of children in our schools who are literally switched-off. When switched on, Ralph can read. He is like a different person. He reads with rhythm and expression in his voice and the stress is gone. Instead of struggling to sound words out, he remembers them or figures them out from context. He uses enough word analysis to unlock the word, and goes on, without breaking his train of thought. He remembers what he reads, and loves it. Brenda, when "on," slows down a bit and thinks. Her voice is less animated, but more intelligent. She can remember more details, and grasps better the intent of the author. She is relearning to print and write correctly, and is beginning to be able to spell by sound and syllable instead of always memorizing. She can get her own thoughts down on paper with accuracy and fluency.

Ralph and Brenda have been switched-on and they are now ready to learn. Did they remind you of anyone? Ralph is like Brain Left and Brenda is like Brain Right. Ralph, like Brain Left, is trying to learn with the Left Hemisphere of his brain and is blocking the Right for some reason. He is trying to follow the rules, read the sounds, remember the words, and hear the story, all at the same time, but he can't. Brain Left can only do one thing at a time. Brenda, like Brain Right, gets the melody of the language and recognizes sight words, but the Left Hemisphere, which processes languages and phonological elements, is switched off. There is little storage and organization of information.

TRADITIONAL EDUCATIONAL PROCEDURES

Traditional educational procedures would attempt to train Ralph's visual memory and Brenda's auditory language recall. With luck and persistence, it is possible that they would improve and spontaneously function at higher levels of achievement. But, in most cases, training a switched-off brain means teaching a Hemisphere of the brain to compensate and perform functions that it does not do easily, and it is seldom done successfully.

Americans seem to have an undying faith in materials and software to solve the literacy problem. Millions of taxpayers' dollars have been spent on reading systems, machines, and computer technology, while ignoring the human machine for which these were all intended. American educators tend to try to change the child to fit the materials, compounding the problem, instead of understanding how people can learn better and more successfully.

Perhaps it is human nature to persist in a behavior, long after failure has been assured. There is the often repeated story about the experiment at U.C.L.A. where giant mazes were built to replicate those run by rats in laboratory experiments. College students were to run the mazes in search of money and their performance compared to that of rats in search of cheese. The students quickly learned the task, and there was no significant difference in their performance and that of the rats, until the extinction part of the experiment. When the rewards were removed, the rats stopped looking for the cheese, but the students kept on running those mazes for that "green stuff."

All of us who have taught are guilty of "running mazes." We have succeeded with a method with one child or class, and we are convinced that it should work with another child or class as well. If it doesn't work, it is not the method. Something is wrong with the learner. Each day, week, and year, we keep on hammering away, and the slightest success only reinforces us to keep on the course of ultimate failure.

FRED, A TRUE "DYSLEXIC."

It takes a dramatic challenge to shake us loose from "the failure syndrome" described above. I was fortunate enough to find the challenge in Fred. Fred taught me that most of what I thought I knew about reading and learning had to be reprogrammed. Here, after ten years in the field, I had met a true "dyslexic." Fred could not read at all. He could not remember more than twenty first grade words, though age twenty-six and a high school graduate. Fred was handsome and healthy and showed no apparent physical signs of his disability. He was a charming conversationalist and wanted to learn to read and write very badly. He developed a "faith" in me and agreed to try my methods.

We commenced with the auditory-visual-kinesthetic-tactile approach we had developed emphasizing phonetic blending of letter sounds. Fred learned to sound out stories such as "the fat cat is in the bag" and learned a first grade sight vocabulary through kinesthetic-tactile tracing. He accomplished this in six months, and he was ecstatic.

Then we hit the snag. Fred stopped improving. There was no transfer from our training to the printed page. Children who receive our training take the success and the skills and start to perform at school. Parents' changed perceptions of their children create an atmosphere and an Energy for a new positive attitude about learning. Fred, however, had nothing but twenty years of failure and could not change his self-concept.

Fred is typical of over fifty percent of all problem learners in that he is right-handed, but left-eyed. Crossed-dominance suggests a cause for confusion due to lack of neurological organization. Our visual training program using Getman's bilateral patterning was prescribed for Fred and he completed the program successfully. The improvement in reading and writing, experienced by most children, did not materialize for Fred. Why weren't our methods working for him? They worked for other severe learning disability cases. Was Fred that different from others? Was there some emotional blockage that prevented learning? I was determined to find the solution to Fred's reading problem.

GRACE, A STROKE VICTIM

About that time, I met Grace, who provided me with insight to help Fred. Grace was seventy-two and had had a stroke. Apparently rehabilitated in every way, she could not read and was heartbroken. An avid reader before the illness and president of a book club, she wished to regain this part of her social life. The family asked me if I could help. Money was no object. I said I would try. I would attempt our bilateral integration and retrain Grace in sound-sight relationships so she could figure out words. Soon she was reading much better. She knew the words as "sight" words. She could read words in lists, but she could not read printed language from a book beyond the fifth grade level. Knowing the etiology of Grace's disability, trauma to the left brain, made the role of each Hemisphere in reading so very obvious.

Fred was not using his Right Brain because focusing his Left Brain required all his attention. He had taught himself to "zero in" and screen out all information except the letter-by-letter decoding that he believed was reading. Grace, with many brain cells destroyed in the Left Brain by her stroke, was reading with only the Right Brain and was unable to process complex verbal materials or decode words phonetically.

Edu-Kinesthetics switched on Fred so that he is now reading Grade Three materials after a year of instruction. Grace learned to focus her attention so that her reading improved to Grade Six level. (I probably learned more from Grace than she learned from me!) The key for Fred was to be able to relax, to back off and trust himself instead of trying so hard. Edu-Kinesthetics gave him enough success that he was able to break his old habits. The key for Grace was to be able to slow down, focus her attention, and relearn to listen to the surface structure of the language.

Edu-Kinesthetics gets people balanced and switched on

before they learn and keeps them balanced while they learn. It is safe and simple. All you need to do is know Brain Right and Brain Left and pay attention to your student.

Edu-Kinesthetics teaches you to maximize a student's potential by eliminating blockages and avoiding stress which interferes with learning. Its premise is that most learning problems are self-imposed, unintentionally. A child, trying to do what is asked of him, switches off and soon makes it a habit.

Pretend that you see Brain Left and Brain Right reading the same selection in front of you. Brain Right has no Left Hemisphere, and Brain Left has no Right If only Brain Left could read a bit faster and with more meaning in his voice. Brain Right just says the words she knows, and keeps getting stumped by the little words like "in" and "on" and says "was" for "saw." If only the two of them could fuse together and share their own special talents. All at once they seem to melt into one and the reading becomes natural, accurate, and alive like actual conversational language. Each side does its share in the information processing, and the thought of the writer is communicated to the reader and the listener.

IN SUMMARY

1. Edu-Kinesthetics is used to both diagnose blockages in the learning process and to remediate learning disabilities by unjamming the circuits.

2. Movement and body awareness is a part of the learning process, to not only build Left Brain dominance, but to integrate the Right Brain into every experience.

3. Blocking the Right Brain inhibits reading and writing. These skills must become automatic like breathing and digestion, and is ultimately a Right Brain function.

4. To assure an integrated and balanced learning experience, one must be aware of:
   a) The midline of the body.
   b) Fluid movement of eyes, hands, and body.
   c) Cross-motor patterning.
   d) Expressive language skills and overt body language.
   e) Energy flow through the neck.
   f) Awareness of the body while thinking.
   g) The inevitability of successful learning.
   h) Emphasis on the present. The past and future must not

detract from the joy of present success.
   i) Emphasis on the process. The product will take care of itself.
   j) Acceptance of responsibility for one's own growth.
5. Edu-Kinesthetics helps to switch on a high level of vital awareness in the healthy learner. It is not:
   a) A panacea.
   b) A substitute for appropriate medical, dental, and vision care.
   c) A substitute for excellence in teaching and a warm and loving home environment.

CHAPTER XI
E-K IN ACTION

THE POSEIDON SCHOOL

"So E-K works with dyslexics at your reading clinics. But what research and experience do you have that proves E-K will work in the classroom?" Such was the response of interested parents and educators who heard about our program.

Convinced that E-K can work for anyone, if properly implemented, I designed a program for the Poseidon School in Los Angeles. This pilot study would provide data to indicate whether Edu-Kinesthetics is a viable educational alternative.

The Poseidon School is a private special education school serving approximately sixty youngsters of Jr. and Sr. High School age. These students are referred to Poseidon School by school districts, courts, and the private sector. Most have given up on the idea of being able to learn. Believing themselves to be failures, they are alienated from the world of academics, family, and often friends.

AN EDUCATIONAL PHILOSOPHY

Believing that successful living requires a total atmosphere and environment for growth, our program sought to initiate changes at Poseidon first from the staff's philosophical point of view, before introducing it to the students. More than a course of study, or a teaching machine, or just another gimmick, E-K is a way of life. Implementing E-K, then, would require that it be internalized into the belief system, however subtly, of all personnel involved in the program, from Directors, counselors, and teachers to parents, secretaries, and custodial staff. When there is a belief that growth in a school is possible, then all who work there will work subconsciously to actualize that belief.

STAFF DEVELOPMENT

The program, as presented to Poseidon School, sought first to "switch on" the entire staff in a group seminar. During December of 1980, in an all day, eight hour experience, staff members were exposed to all aspects of E-K, as if they were the children in a "hands-on," workshop environment of fun, discovery, and introspection. The goal was to offer the possibilities of E-K in the classroom, without requiring it by administrative fiat. We hoped a teacher would come forward who would want to attempt E-K on a provisional basis with her class. All enjoyed the seminar and saw purpose and value in the information provided. Fortunately, one teacher volunteered to participate in a pilot program.

The staff met the following week and was told by the director that E-K would be introduced in one classroom during the Spring semester, with the possibility of a wider application in the future. All were invited to observe and experiment with those aspects of the program with which they were comfortable. They were told that Dr. Dennison would provide consultation services and in-service training for the teacher, parents, and teaching assistants of the pilot study class throughout the semester.

ACCOUNTABILITY

To document the changes, if any, the Peabody Picture Vocabulary Test, a test of vocabulary word recognition, was administered to the 19 students involved in the study as it began in January of 1981. The score on this test can be converted into an Intelligence Quotient, a number used in this case for purposes of measuring changes. A growth of 7 or more points would be considered indicative of significant change occurring during the initial five months of the program.

THE CLASSROOM

Lois Fabiano, the teacher of the class, started with Edu-Kinesthetics by following the "right brain" prescript that "the whole is more than the sum of its parts." She knew that a philosophical change must take place first, before the students would believe that they were capable of learning, loving, and growing. She started with herself and her teaching assistant, balancing each other, thinking positive thoughts, and assuming an attitude of unconditional love and openness to growth.

Lois held class discussions about E-K, always making it clear that participation was completely voluntary. One at a time, more and more students became involved, asking questions and making suggestions. Slowly the students were guided to awareness of the following:

1. Muscle testing of each other.
2. The physical room environment.
3. The effects of colors, foods, and posture.
4. The relationship of cross-crawling and learning.
5. The relaxing benefits of natural sounds and music played at slower tempos.

THE STUDENTS

The students removed pictures and decorations which weakened them, and brought in visually balancing items for their eyes. Curtains were made by the teacher to provide a psychological and visible barrier to the harshness of the outside world. Those who so desired did aerobic cross-crawling to music outside the classroom in the playground. Plastic furniture was eliminated and replaced with wooden tables, which were found to be better conductors of energy, and more comfortable. An aquarium was purchased so that both the sounds of water and the presence of life pervaded the room. A meeting of the parents was held one evening to explain the program and demonstrate E-K's applications. The response was overwhelmingly positive and enthusiastic.

RESULTS

A dynamic of helping, touching, and loving grew in the class as the weeks went by. A respect for the room, its content, and its sanctity as a place to share and learn, developed. Ben, a severe dysgraphic, who could neither write very well nor spell, was guided by his teacher and classmates to correct learning habits. Napoleon, a hyperactive boy, six feet tall and usually disruptive, became a wealth of information on metaphysical matters and offered his own interpretations of what was happening, most of which was quite helpful to the class.

Students were still active and boisterous but there was less anger and hostility, and each person respected the "space" of the other. Visitors noticed a difference immediately and asked what was happening in the room. Students listened better, both to each other and to the teacher, and grades on weekly assignments improved.

In June of 1981, the Peabody Picture Vocabulary Test was re-administered. As a measure of receptive language ability, correlating highly with other predictive measures of academic success, the scores reflect the changes E-K made on the lives of these students.

Of the original 19 participants, two left the class leaving 17 students for the post test. Of these 17, 11 had improved scores, one stayed the same, and 5 went down. Eight of the changes, up and down, were of only 2 to 4 points and were, therefore, not statistically significant. However, seven of the students improved their scores from 7 to 14 points, suggesting a significant change in one's awareness and openness to learning. (See Figure 1)

POSEIDON SCHOOL
EDU-KINESTHETICS PILOT STUDY
PEABODY PICTURE VOCABULARY TEST

Student	Pre-test 1/81	Post-test 6/81	Change
A	106	109	+3
B	109	left	
C	114	114	same
D	103	100	−3
E	108	110	+2
F	89	left	
G	77	87	+10
H	98	111	+13
I	100	97	−3
J	105	94	−11
K	111	125	+14
L	108	104	−4
M	84	95	+11
N	123	134	+10
O	111	121	+10
P	94	98	+4
Q	101	108	+7
R	79	82	+3

Figure 1. The change in intelligence quotients on a test of receptive language ability showed a trend toward improved scores for eleven out of seventeen students exposed to Edu-Kinesthetics, with seven improving from 7 to 14 points.

Edu-Kinesthetics, when implemented as it was at Poseidon, is a tool to make all learning and growth more successful. When people can work together in a helpful, understanding, and positive way, all things are possible. We have only just begun!

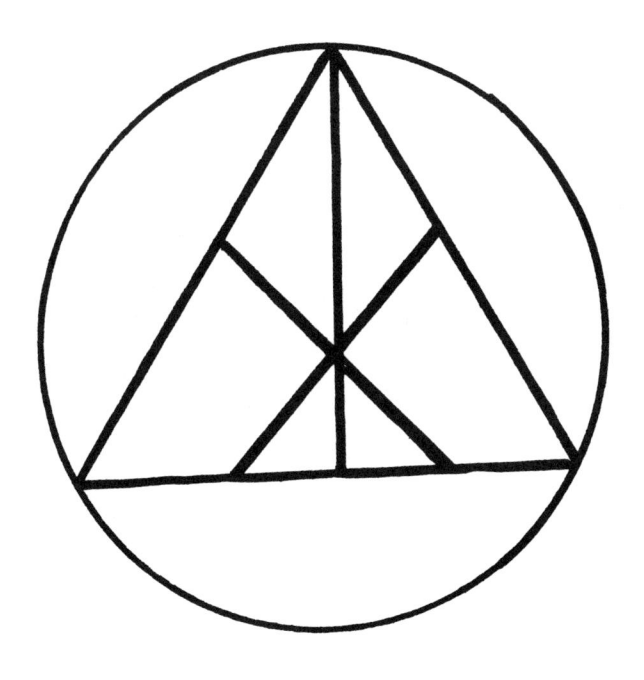

Fig. 2 The Symbol of Edu-Kinesthetics.

OUR SYMBOL

To remember what Edu-Kinesthetics can do for you, let's look at the meaning of our symbol. (See Figure 2) If you meditate upon its meaning in the weeks and months ahead, you will gain renewed insight into the nature of Edu-Kinesthetics.

Our logo shows a pyramid within a circle, with several lines within the pyramid, connecting at a point in the center of the circle. The logo is highly symbolic of all that has been presented in this book.

The circle represents Life and Energy, which is moving, dynamic, and ever-changing. Expressive Energy radiates counterclockwise from the center as we grow. Centering, meditative Energy moves clockwise inward, toward the center as we focus attention. The pyramid attracts Energy from the Universe through its apex, and is grounded to the earth at its base where we experience Life through the senses. The right and left sides of the pyramid symbolize the Right and Left Brain, our two modes of consciousness, connected in the center by the Corpus Collosum. The two brains are interconnected by two little lines which cross its center, and enter each other's sphere of consciousness at the base, symbolizing cross motor patterning. The base of the pyramid represents the visual field, and the central one-third of that line is the midline field where integrated, switched on learning takes place. The line running from base to apex also represents Energy, which must flow through the body and neck in order to keep us balanced and in good posture.

DEFINITION OF TERMS

Applied Kinesiology—Using the science of muscle testing to obtain information from the brain and body.

Balancing—The restoration of Energy flow which may be blocked due to stress.

Edu-kinesthetics—The application of Kinesthetics to the study of Right Brain, Left Brain, and body integration for purposes of eliminating stress and utilizing full Energy potential to facilitate learning.

Muscle Testing—The technique of measuring the relative strength of selected muscles to detect Energy imbalances which may be relevant to educators.

Muscle Weakness—The inability to activate a muscle due to Energy blockage.

Switched-Off—The inhibition of Right or Left Hemisphere, due to stress or "trying" too hard.

Reading—The process of interpreting printed language as one's own active thought process through integration of visual, auditory and body information centers.

Writing—The process of expressing oneself through body movement while maintaining Right Brain-Left Brain balance and coordination.

APPENDIX
EDU-EXERCISES

Included in this section are exercises and activities, not mentioned in the text, which we have found useful in special cases to relieve tension, improve posture and promote hemispheric integration and balance.

1. *Swinging*

   Swinging is excellent to stimulate the sense of balance and motor control. Swing in all positions, faster to excite and slower to relax.

2. *Spinning*

   Spinning provides miraculous effects on both motor development and concentration. It stimulates the vestibular mechanism, a part of the inner ear, which controls balance.

3. *Hanging Upside-Down*

   Inverted positions help direct blood and Energy to the brain. The body can experience a fully extended posture and a sense of weightlessness.

   It is found particularly good for visual problems.

4. *Jumping on a Trampoline*

   Jumping on a trampoline, which provides a rebound into a weightless state, is excellent for both vestibular stimulation and visual proprioception. Stop-motion photography shows the eyes relearning to focus and point.

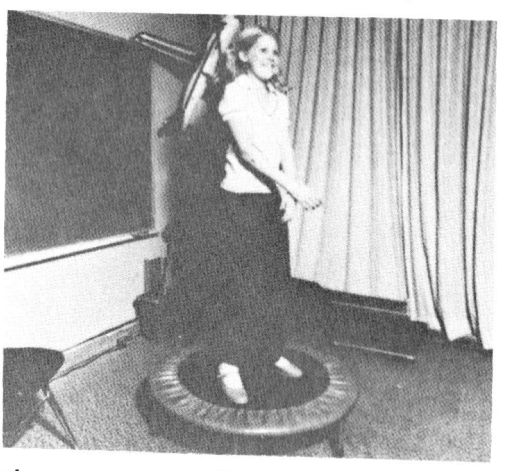

Fig. 1 Jumping on a trampoline enables one to experience the state of weightlessness.

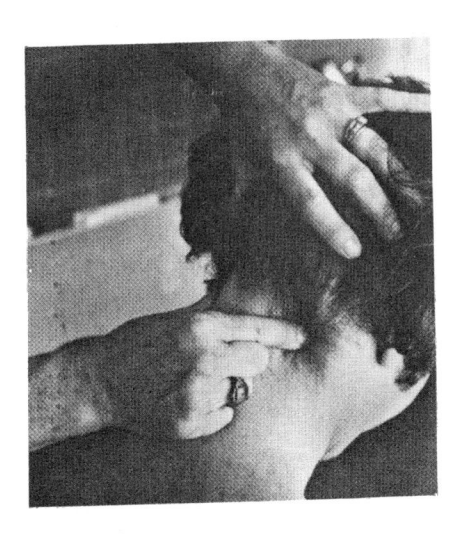

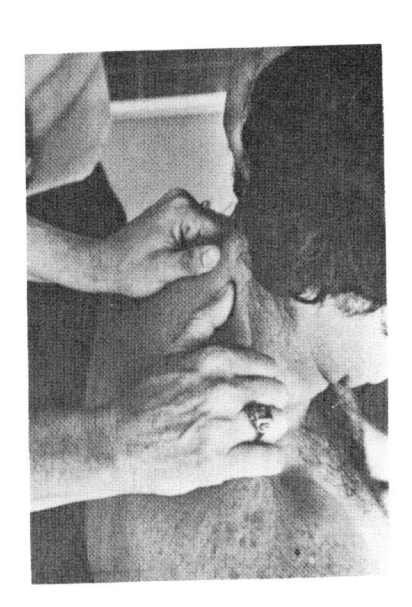

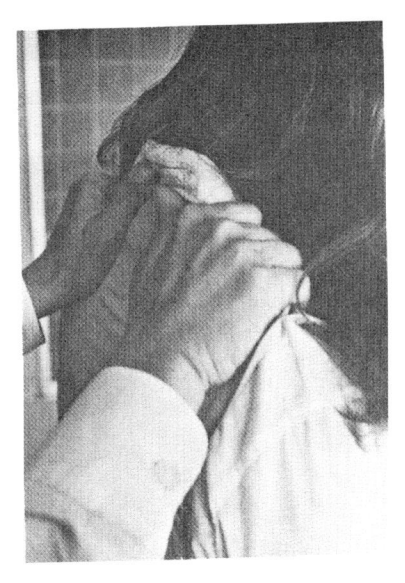

Fig. 3 Tension in the shoulders can be relieved by gripping and squeezing the muscle tissue between the neck and the shoulders.

5. *Massaging*

Massaging relieves tension at every age, and children need massaging just as much as do adults. Particular attention should be paid to the back of the upper neck, where it joins the head. (See Figure 2)

If shoulders look tense or feel hard, squeeze these muscles firmly for about twenty seconds, as tightly as the person will permit, and the tension will melt away. (See Figure 3)

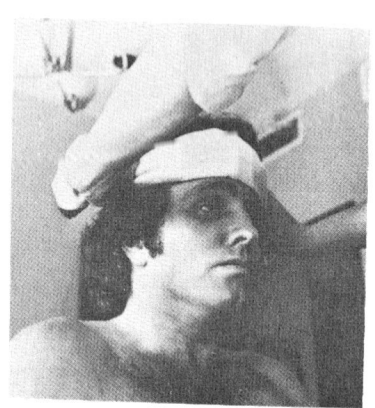

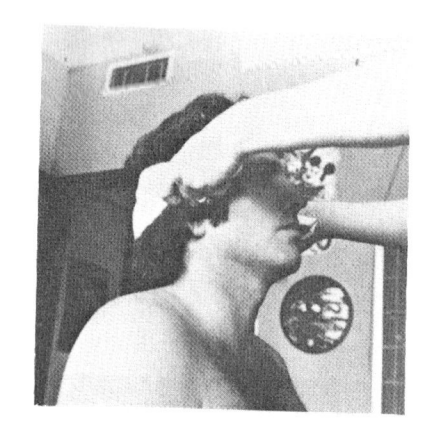

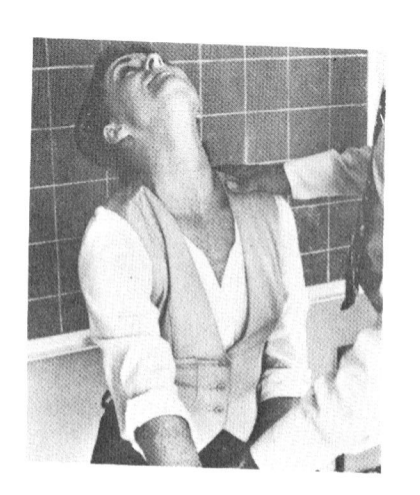

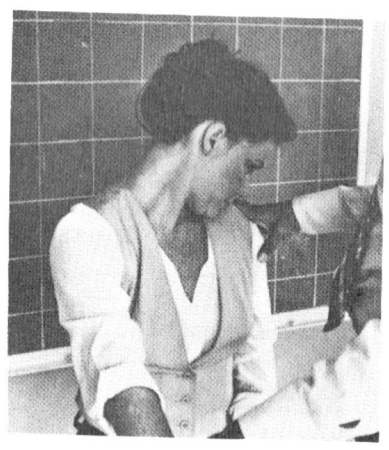

Fig. 5 Relaxation exercises for the neck muscles. Roll the head in complete rotations. Hold wherever there is tension, until it lets go.

6. *Strengthening and Relaxing the Neck*

We exercise and strengthen other muscles of the body, but we take our neck muscles for granted. Resistance exercises, as shown in Figure 4, help to activate the neck muscles so that the neck becomes more responsive to the environment, and a better conductor of Energy. Alternate strengthening exercises with neck rolls as shown in Figure 5. Do not force the neck rolls. Let gravity and Energy do the moving. First, let your head hang forward until all the tension is gone, and slowly rotate the head. do it three times in each direction.

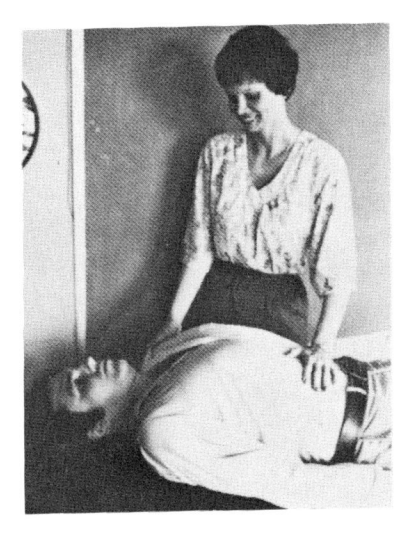

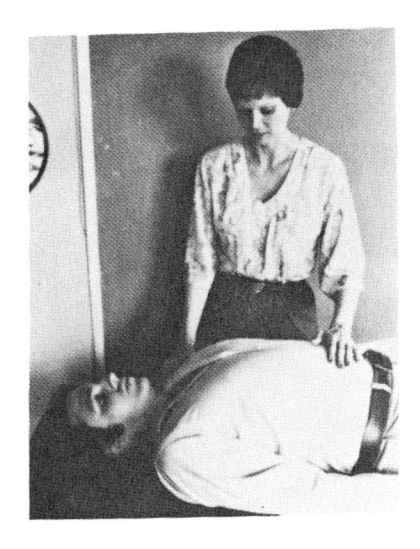

Fig. 6 Incorrect breathing is shallow, into the chest only. Correct breathing fills the entire abdominal cavity upon inhale, as well as the chest.

7. *Breathing Exercises*

Many people do not know how to breathe and block Energy with every breath. Shallow breathing is learned as a "fight or flight" response, and fills the chest only. Some people hold in the stomach to look thin. Correct breathing fills the whole body, from abdomen to upper chest, and sends Energy to every cell of the body. It is easiest to learn lying down on the back. A hand or a book on the abdominal region draws Energy to that area. Note any tension in the body and let it go. Breathe rhythmically, breathing in slowly—1, 2, 3—holding the breath in—1, 2, 3—and exhaling slowly—1, 2, 3. The count may be increased with experience. We breathe through the nostrils for this exercise. (See Figure 6)

BIBLIOGRAPHY

Adler, Ronald B., and Towne, Neil. *Looking Out/Looking In.* New York: Holt, Rinehart and Winston, 1981.
Assagoioli, Roberto. *Psychosynthesis.* New York: Penguin Books, 1976.
Ayres, A. Jean. *Sensory Integration and Learning Disorders.* Los Angeles: Western Psychologist Services, 1973.
Bach, Richard. *Illusions.* U.S.: Delacorte Press, 1977.
Rakan, Paulo. "The Eyes Have It" in *Psychology Today.* Vol 4, No. 11, pp 64-67, 96, April, 1971.
Bandler, Richard and Grinder, John. *Frogs Into Princes.* Moab, Utah: Real People Press, 1979.
Blakeslee, Thomas R. *The Right Brain.* Garden City, N.Y.: Doubleday, 1980.
Buzan, Tony. *Use Both Sides of Your Brain.* New York: E.P. Dutton, 1974.
Delacato, Carl H. *The Diagnosis and Treatment of Speech and Reading Problems.* Springfield, Illinois: Charles C. Thomas, 1963.
Dennison, Paul Ehrlich. Covert Speech and Beginning Reading Achievement. Unpublished Doctoral Dissertation, University of Southern California Graduate School, 1975.
Diamond, John. B.K. *Behavioral Kinesiology.* New York: Harper and Row, 1979.
Eastcett, Michael J. *The Silent Path: An Introduction to Meditation.* New York: Weiser, 1969.
Edwards, Betty. *Drawing on the Right Side of the Brain.* Los Angeles: J.P. Tarcher, Inc., 1979.
Ferguson, Marilyn. *The Brain Revolution.* New York: Taplinger Publishing Company, 1973.
Ferguson, Marilyn. *The Aquarian Conspiracy.* Los Angeles: J.P. Tarcher, Inc., 1980.
Green, Elmer and Alyce. *Beyond Biofeedback.* U.S.: Delacorte Press, 1977.
Joy, W. Brugh. *Joy's Way.* Los Angeles: J.P. Tarcher, Inc., 1979.
Murphy, J. *The Power of the Subconscious Mind.* New Jersey: Prentiss, 1963.
Myers, Patricia I. *Methods of Learning Disorders.* New York: John Wiley and Sons, Inc., 1969.
Osman, Betty B. *Learning Disabilities, A Family Affair.* New York: Random House, 1979.

Ornstein, Robert E. "Right and Left Thinking" in *Psychology Today*. Vol 6, No. 12, pp 86-92, May. 1973.

Ostrander, Sheila and Schroeder, Lynn. *Superlearning*. New York: Dell Publishing Co., 1979.

Oyle, Irving. *The New American Medicine Show*. Santa Cruz, California: Unity Press, 1979.

Pelletier, Kenneth R. *Mind as Healer, Mind as Slayer*. New York: Delta Press, 1977.

Rama, Ballantine and Weinstock. *Yoga and Psychotherapy*. Glenview, Illinois: Himalayan Institute, 1967.

Shinn, Florence. *The Game of Life and How to Play it*. Brooklyn: Gerald Richard, 1941.

Solan, Harold A. *Psychology of Reading Difficulties*. Selected Academic Reading, 1968.

Spiegel, John P. and Machetka, Pavel. *Messages of the Body*. New York: The Free Press, 1974.

Thie, John F. *Touch for Health*. Marina del Rey, California: DeVorsse Co., 1973.

Virshup, Evelyn. *Right Brain People in a Left Brain World*. Los Angeles: The Guild of Tutors Press, 1978.

Walthers, David S. *Applied Kinesiology, The Advanced Approach to Chiropractic*. Pueblo, Colorado: Systems DC, 1976.

Weiner, Harold. *Eyes OK, I'm OK*. San Rafael, California: Academic Therapy Publications, 1977.

INDEX

Applied Kinesiology, 11, 31, 112
Auditory Integration, see Integration
Auditory Learner, see Learning Types
Auricular Exercise, 79; see also Earedness

Balance, 13, 15-16, 29, 32, 48-49; see also Balance Dimensions
Balancing, Muscles, 32, 36, 112; Energy 28, 49; For Stress, 32-34
Being, 56
Bennett Reflex, 31
Bilateral Integration, see Integration
Bilateral Movements, 35, 40
Biofeedback, 31
Brainedness, 61-64
Brain, 79-80
Brain Left, 76-78, 100, 103
Brain Right, 76-78, 100, 103
Breathing Exercises, 116-117

CLEMS, 61
Color, 24
Convergence Exercises, see Eye Exercises
Corpus Callosum, 80
Counterclockwise Motion, 94-96
Creeping and Crawling, 40-47, 68
Cross-Crawling, 35, 37; see also Cross-Dominant, 60-61, 101
Cross-Motor Patterning, see Cross-Crawling
Culture, Modern American, 14-15, 24-29

Delacato, Carl H., 36
Deltoid, 17-19, 23, 25
Dennison's Laterality Checklist, 75
Dominance, 36, 57-58; see also Lateral Dominance, Cross-Dominance
Dominant Brain, test for, 60
Dyslexia, 12, 35-37, 40, 101

Earedness, 70-73
Ears, see Earedness
Edu-Exercises 113-117
Edu-Kinesthetics, 11-13, 14-16, 24-26, 31, 32-34, 48, 50, 57, 61, 66, 89, 93, 103-104, 105-106, 112; see Movement Re-education
E-K Symbol, 111
Emotional Response, 32
Emotional Stress Release, 32
Energy, 11, 14-19, 24, 27, 36; see also Life Force
Energy Balance, see Balancing, Energy
Energy Blockage, 17, 24, 26
Energy Field, 15; see also Lifespace
Energy Imbalances, 18
Enjoying, 56
Environment, 28
Environmental Factor, 25
Extinction Conditioning, 43
Eyedness, 57-60
Eye Exercises, 68
Eye Movements, Binocular, 64

Feeling, 56
Fight or Flight, 30-32, 34
Food Testing, 26-27
Frontal Eminences, 32-34

Gestalt, 36
Goodheart, George, 31; see also Applied Kinesiology
Gravity, 49-50
Green, Elmer, 31

Handedness, 36, 57-60, 93
Hanging upside-down, see Edu-Exercises
Harnack, Dick, 35
Hemispheres, 36, 40, 80, 83-87; see also Right Brain, Left Brain
Hemispheric Specialization, 94
Homolateral Crawling. example of, 43-44

Homolateral Movements, 40; see also Homolateral Crawling, example of Homolateral Stage, 43
Integration, 36, 40, 58; Auditory, 71-72; Bilateral, 58, 102; Visual, 66
Intention, 17
Indicator Muscle, 17, 25

Jumping on a trampoline, see Edu-Exercises

Kinesiology, 11

Language, 73-74
Lateral Dominance, 57-75; see also Dominance
Latissimus Dorsi, 17, 19, 22, 27
Lazy 8, 94-96
Learning Disabilities, 16
Learning Types, 88-89;
Left-Brain, 36-37, 43, 57-58, 61, 71-72, 83, 87, 88, 89; see also Hemispheres
Left-handedness, 60
Letters, 94-96
Life Force, 50; see also Energy
Lifespace, 15, 24, 28; see also Energy Field
Limbic System, 30
Love, 13, 16, 24

Massage, for eyes, 68; see also Edu-Exercises
Meditation, 31
Midline, 86-87
Mixed-Dominant, see also Cross-Dominant
Movement Re-education, 47, 53; see also Edu-Kinesthetics
Muscles, 16-18; see also Balancing, Muscles
Muscle Testing, 14-18
Muscle Weakness, 112
Music, 25-26

Nature, 28
Neck, Importance of, 49; Strengthening and relaxing, 116
Negativity, effects of, 27, 28-29

Neurological Organizaton, see Lateral Dominance

Orton, Samuel T., 36
Ostrander, Sheila, 26

Pectoralis Major Clavicular, 17, 19, 21, 32
People, effects of, 28-29
Plastics, effects of, 28
Poseidon School, 105-109
Postural Analysis, 55
Posture, 12, 48;
  muscle test for, 50-53, 55;
  muscle test for writing posture, 98
Psycho-Motor Training, 11
Pursuits, see Eye Exercises

Range of Motion, 17-18
Reading, 58, 99-104, 112
Right-Brain, 36-37, 43, 57-58, 61, 71-72, 83, 88-89, 93; see also Hemispheres
Rotations, see Eye Exercises

Schroeder, Lynn, see Ostrander, Sheila
Self-concept, 32, 34
Sitting, 53
Sound, 26
Spelling, 58
Spinning, see Edu-Exercises
Stimulus-Response, 29
Strenghthening, 13, 16, 32
Stress, effects of, 30-32;
  Balancing for, 32-34, 87
Subconscious, 58
Superlearning, 26
Supraspinatus, 17, 19-20
Survival Instinct, 31
Swinging, see Edu-Exercises
Switching-off, 16-18, 24, 43, 48;
  at midline, 86;
  Visual System, 64-66;
  Writing, 96-98, 112
Switching-on, 16-17, 43;
  Ears, 73, 79
  Visual System, 66
  Writing, 98

121

Television, effects of, 28
Thie, John F., D.C., 11, 18, 32; see Touch for Health
Touch For Health, 18, 35; see John F. Thie, D.C.
Touching, 14-15, 18
2-2-2 Technique, 18

Visual Field, 64
Visual Integration, test for, 66; see also Integration
Visual Learner, see Learning Types
Visualizing, 55-56
Visual Switching-off, see Switching-off

Walther, David S., 68
Weaken, 16, 50, 53
Words, power of, 27
Writing, 53, 58, 93-98, 112
Writing Analysis, 91-98

Yoga, 31; for eyes, 68

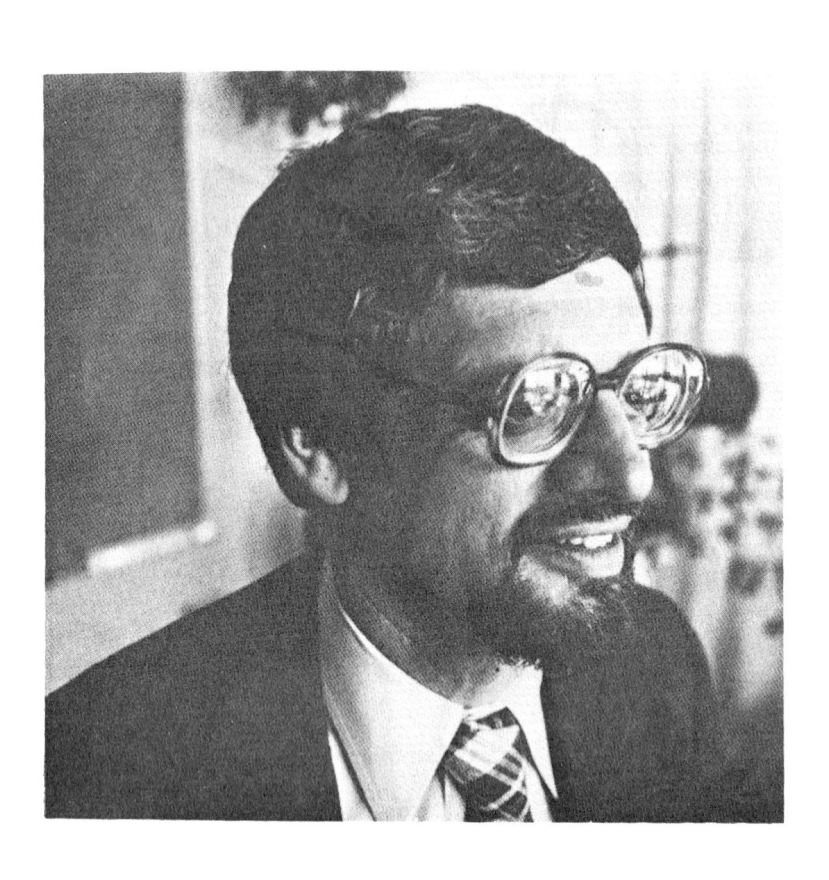

ABOUT THE AUTHOR:

Paul E. Dennison, Ph.D., has been an educator for all of his professional life. He is the creator of the Edu-Kinesthetics and Brain Gym processes, and a pioneer in applied brain research. His discoveries are based upon an understanding of the interdependence of physical development, language acquisition, and academic achievement. This perspective grew out of his background in curriculum development and experimental psychology at the University of Southern California, where he was granted a Doctorate in Education for his research in beginning reading achievement and its relationship to thinking. For nineteen years, Dr. Dennison served as director of the Valley Remedial Group Learning Centers in Southern California, helping children and adults turn their difficulties into successful growth. He is the author of twelve books and manuals, including *Switching On: A Guide to Edu-Kinesthetics*.

The following are some of the courses offered by the Educational Kinesiology Foundation, P.O. Box 3396, Ventura, CA 93006-3396 • (800) 356-2109

- **BRAIN GYM®** - 24 hours, consisting of Part I, **The Lateral Brain** and Part II, **The Whole Brain**
This Brain Gym course offers an in depth experience of hemispheric integration through Dennison Laterality Repatterning and 23 Brain Gym activities that relate to whole-brain functioning. A process for achieving deeper structural integration through Three-Dimension Repatterning is also included. The effects of incomplete development of laterality, centering, and focus on posture, reading, writing, spelling, and memory are identified and balanced. Course Manual: *Brain Gym® Handbook* by Dennison and Dennison.

- **EDU-KINESTHETICS IN DEPTH: The Seven Dimensions of Intelligence** - 32 hours
Learn and practice the Edu-Kinesthetics principles through an individualized educational model. Receive hands-on experience with seven dimensions of body intelligence, focusing on how each can support or block the learning process. Other areas covered in the course include: appropriate goal setting, learning theory, and growth-oriented communication. Course Manual: *Edu-Kinesthetics In Depth: The Seven Dimensions of Intelligence*. Prerequisite: Brain Gym, Parts I & II.

- **BRAIN GYM TEACHER PRACTICUM** - 32 hours
A certification course qualifying the student to teach Brain Gym. Completion of this course provides the graduate with specific skills for teaching the Brain Gym course. This workshop prepares the instructor to represent the Foundation in the community. Course Manual: *Teacher Practicum Manual*. Prerequisite: Edu-Kinesthetics in Depth.

EDU-KINESTHETICS PUBLICATIONS

U.S. Funds

SWITCHING ON by Dr. Paul E. Dennison $12.95
EDU-K FOR KIDS by Dennison & Dennison $12.00
PERSONALIZED WHOLE BRAIN INTEGRATION by Dennison & Dennison $15.95
BRAIN GYM® by Dennison & Dennison ....$ 8.00
BRAIN GYM®, **Teacher's Edition** by Dennison & Dennison $16.95
BRAIN GYM® **SURFER** by Hinsley & Conley ....$ 6.00
EDU-KINESTHETICS IN DEPTH. $29.95
INTEGRATED MOVEMENTS (audio tape) $12.00

Mail your order to: **Edu-Kinesthetics, Inc.,** Post Office Box 3396, Ventura, California 93006-3396 U.S.A. Telephone or fax order with VISA/MC: Telephone (805) 650-3303 • FAX (805) 650-0524

Prices do not include postage and handling charges (approximately $1.50 per title), which will be added to your order. California residents must add sales tax. Quantity discounts available. Allow three weeks delivery time.